HANDBOOK OF DIFFERENTIAL DIAGNOSIS IN INTERNAL MEDICINE:
MEDICAL BOOK OF LISTS

HANDBOOK OF DIFFERENTIAL DIAGNOSIS IN INTERNAL MEDICINE: *MEDICAL BOOK OF LISTS*

a mosby handbook

NORTON J. GREENBERGER, MD
Peter T. Bohan Professor and Chairman
Department of Medicine
University of Kansas Medical Center
Kansas City, Kansas

MARK S. BERNTSEN MD
Co-Chief Resident
Department of Medicine
University of Kansas Medical Center
Kansas City, Kansas

DAVID K. JONES, MD
Co-Chief Resident
Department of Medicine
University of Kansas Medical Center
Kansas City, Kansas

VINOD N. VELAKATURI, MD
Co-Chief Resident
Department of Medicine
University of Kansas Medical Center
Kansas City, Kansas

FIFTH EDITION

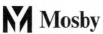

Mosby
A Harcourt Health Sciences Company
St. Louis   London   Philadelphia   Sydney   Toronto

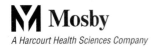
Mosby
A Harcourt Health Sciences Company

Publisher: Laura DeYoung
Editor: Simon Pritchard
Developmental Editor: Pui F. Szeto
Project Manager: Carol Sullivan Weis
Designer: Jen Marmarinos
Manufacturing Manager: Dave Graybill

Mosby, Inc.
11830 Westline Industrial Drive
St. Louis, Missouri 63146

0-323-00131-9

01 02/9 8 7 6 5 4 3

To my wife, Joan Narcus Greenberger, *for her superb redactory efforts in reviewing all the tables in all five editions of this textbook.*

PREFACE

The fifth edition of this book expands on the format of the first four editions, which have been well received by medical students, house officers, and faculty and for which the authors are most appreciative.

Two of the most important considerations in the practice of internal medicine are the formulation of the differential diagnosis and the recognition of precise criteria on which to base a specific diagnosis. We have written this book because we believe that there is a need for a reasonably brief treatise that deals primarily with differential diagnosis. The book is a direct outgrowth of morning report sessions at the University of Kansas Medical Center. At these sessions, cases are presented as "unknowns" and resident physicians are asked to develop a differential diagnosis and also to indicate the specific criteria necessary to establish various diagnoses. This book, which contains over 300 lists, is a selective distillation of topics covered at morning report exercises. As such, the book is not a substitute for standard textbooks of medicine. Rather, it is viewed as a quick reference to key questions that may arise on ward rounds or at conference. The fifth edition has been extensively revised with 35 new tables and 45 revised tables.

Several individuals have made great contributions to this book, and we thank Shirley Sears and Ruth Stricklen for their preparation of the manuscript.

Norton J. Greenberger
Mark S. Berntsen
David K. Jones
Vinod N. Velakaturi

Contents

II.   ENDOCRINOLOGY—METABOLISM

III. GASTROENTEROLOGY

IV.   HEMATOLOGY—ONCOLOGY

V. INFECTIOUS DISEASE

VI. NEPHROLOGY

VII. PULMONARY DISEASE

VIII.   CLINICAL IMMUNOLOGY AND RHEUMATOLOGY

IX. NEUROLOGY

X. DERMATOLOGY

XI. ACQUIRED IMMUNODEFICIENCY SYNDROME (AIDS)

HANDBOOK OF DIFFERENTIAL DIAGNOSIS IN INTERNAL MEDICINE:
MEDICAL BOOK OF LISTS

CHAPTER I

Cardiology

I-1   INNOCENT MURMURS

  I. Patients in whom innocent murmurs are more likely to occur
- A. Children and adolescents
- B. Pregnant women
- C. Anxious persons
- D. Funnel-breasted or flat-chested persons
- E. Persons with the straight back syndrome
- F. Hyperthyroid and anemic persons

  II. Types of innocent murmurs

Innocent murmurs may be classified as follows:
- A. Completely innocent
  1. Cervical venous hum
  2. Supraclavicular arterial bruit
  3. Still's murmur
  4. Mammary souffle
  5. Ejection systolic murmur in the pulmonary area
  6. Innocent abdominal murmurs
- B. Relatively innocent
  1. Early systolic murmur
  2. Pulmonary systolic murmur with high output states (hemic murmur)

I-2   CAUSES OF SPLITTING OF THE SECOND HEART SOUND

  I. Delayed pulmonic closure

Delayed electrical activation of the right ventricle
- A. Complete RBBB (proximal type)
- B. Left ventricular paced beats
- C. Left ventricular ectopic beats

  II. Prolonged right ventricular mechanical systole
- A. Acute massive pulmonary embolus
- B. Pulmonary hypertension with right heart failure
- C. Pulmonic stenosis with intact septum (moderate to severe)

  III. Decreased impedance of the pulmonary vascular bed (increased hang-out)
- A. Normotensive atrial septal defect
- B. Idiopathic dilatation of the pulmonary artery
- C. Pulmonic stenosis (mild)
- D. Atrial septal defect, postoperative (70%)

  IV. Early aortic closure

Shortened left ventricular mechanical systole (LVET)
- A. Mitral regurgitation
- B. Ventricular septal defect

Continued

I-2 CAUSES OF SPLITTING OF THE SECOND HEART SOUND—*cont'd*

   V. Delayed aortic closure (AES)
      Delayed electrical activation of the left ventricle
      A. Complete LBBB (proximal type)
      B. Right ventricular paced beats
      C. Right ventricular ectopic beats
      D. Reversed splitting S_2
  VI. Prolonged left ventricular mechanical systole
      A. Complete LBBB (peripheral type)
      B. Left ventricular outflow tract obstruction
      C. Hypertensive cardiovascular disease
      D. Arteriosclerotic heart disease
         1. Chronic ischemic heart disease
         2. Angina pectoris
 VII. Decreased impedance of the systemic vascular bed (increased hang-out)
      A. Poststenotic dilatation of the aorta secondary to aortic stenosis or insufficiency
      B. Patent ductus arteriosus
VIII. Early pulmonic closure
      Early electrical activation of the right ventricle
      A. Wolff-Parkinson-White syndrome, type B

RBBB, Right bundle-branch block; *AES,* audible expiratory splitting; *LVET,* left ventricular ejection time; *LBBB,* left bundle-branch block.

From Perloff JK. In Braunwald E: *Heart disease: A textbook of cardiovascular medicine,* ed 4, Philadelphia, 1992, WB Saunders, pp. 46-48.

I-3 CAUSES OF SINGLE SECOND HEART SOUND

     I. Tetralogy of Fallot
    II. Truncus and pseudotruncus arteriosus
   III. Very severe pulmonary valvular stenosis (occasional case)
   IV. Tricuspid atresia
    V. Aortic stenosis (occasional case)
   VI. Left bundle branch block (occasional case)
  VII. Age over 45 years (variable)
 VIII. Eisenmenger's VSD
   IX. Severe semilunar valve disease
    X. Any of the causes of reversed splitting of second heart sound
   XI. One of the sounds inaudible (e.g., emphysema or obesity)

I-4   PHYSIOLOGIC CLASSIFICATION OF CONTINUOUS MURMURS

I. Continuous murmurs due to rapid blood flow
   A. Venous hum
   B. Mammary souffle
   C. Hemangioma
   D. Hyperthyroidism
   E. Acute alcoholic hepatitis
   F. Hyperemia of neoplasm (hepatoma, renal cell carcinoma, Paget's disease)

II. Continuous murmurs due to high-to-low pressure shunts
   A. Systemic artery to pulmonary artery (patent ductus arteriosus, aortopulmonary window, truncus arteriosus, pulmonary atresia, anomalous left coronary, bronchiectasis, sequestration of the lung)
   B. Systemic artery to right heart (ruptured sinus of Valsalva, coronary artery fistula)
   C. Left-to-right atrial shunting (Lutembacher's syndrome, mitral atresia plus atrial septal defect)
   D. Venovenous shunts (anomalous pulmonary veins, portosystemic shunts)
   E. A-V fistula (systemic or pulmonic)

III. Continuous murmurs secondary to localized arterial obstruction
   A. Coarctation of the aorta
   B. Branch pulmonary stenosis
   C. Carotid occlusion
   D. Celiac mesenteric occlusion
   E. Renal occlusion
   F. Femoral occlusion
   G. Coronary occlusion

From Myers JD: The mechanisms and significances of continuous murmurs. In Leon DF, Shaver JA: *Physiologic principles of heart sounds and murmurs,* monograph 46, New York, 1975, American Heart Association, p. 202. As printed in Hurst JW et al (eds): *The heart,* ed 8, New York, 1994, American Heart Association, p. 307.

I-5   MECHANISMS OF CONTINUOUS MURMURS

I. Connections between aorta and pulmonary artery
II. Arteriovenous fistulas
III. Turbulent flow in arteries
IV. Turbulent flow in veins
V. Communication between left and right atrium
VI. Rapid blood flow

I-6   GUIDELINES FOR THE DIAGNOSIS OF INITIAL ATTACK OF RHEUMATIC FEVER (JONES CRITERIA)

I. Major manifestations
   A. Carditis
   B. Polyarthritis
   C. Chorea
   D. Erythema marginatum
   E. Subcutaneous nodules

II. Minor manifestations
   A. Clinical findings
      1. Arthralgia
      2. Fever
   B. Laboratory findings
      1. Elevated acute phase reactants
      2. Erythrocyte sedimentation rate
      3. C-reactive protein
      4. Prolonged PR interval

III. Supporting evidence of antecedent group A streptococcal infection*
   A. Positive throat culture or rapid streptococcal antigen test
   B. Elevated or rising streptococcal antibody titer

*If supported by evidence of preceding group A streptococcal infection, the presence of two major manifestations or of one major and two minor manifestations indicates a high probability of acute rheumatic fever.

From Special Writing Group: *JAMA* 268(15):2070, 1992.

I-7   CAUSES OF MITRAL REGURGITATION

I. Spontaneous rupture of chordae tendineae
II. Trauma
III. Mitral valve prolapse
IV. Ischemia
V. Myocardial infarction (MI)
VI. Aneurysm of left ventricle involving the mitral annulus
VII. Infective endocarditis
VIII. Congestive cardiomyopathies
IX. IHSS
X. Rheumatic heart disease
XI. SLE
XII. Scleroderma
XIII. Takayasu's arteritis
XIV. Myxomatous degeneration of mitral valve leaflets
XV. Calcified mitral annulus
XVI. Marfan syndrome
XVII. Ehlers-Danlos syndrome
XVIII. Pseudoxanthoma elasticum
XIX. Ankylosing spondylitis
XX. Rheumatoid arthritis
XXI. Congenital (mitral valve clefts, endocardial cushion defects, endocardial fibroelastosis, transposition of the great arteries, anomalous origin of left coronary artery)

SLE, Systemic lupus erythematosus; *IHSS,* idiopathic hypertrophic subaortic stenosis.

I-8   ETIOLOGY OF CHRONIC AND ACUTE AORTIC REGURGITATION*

I. Chronic aortic regurgitation
   A. Rheumatic
   B. Syphilis
   C. Takayasu's arteritis
   D. Annuloaortic ectasia
   E. Heritable disorders of connective tissue
      1. Marfan syndrome
      2. Ehlers-Danlos syndrome
      3. Osteogenesis imperfecta
   F. Congenital heart disease
      1. Bicuspid aortic valve
      2. Interventricular septal defect
      3. Sinus of Valsalva aneurysm
   G. Arthritic diseases
      1. Ankylosing spondylitis
      2. Reiter's syndrome
      3. Rheumatoid arthritis
      4. SLE
      5. Primary antiphospholipid syndrome
   H. Cystic medial necrosis of aorta
   I. Hypertension
   J. Arteriosclerosis
   K. Myxomatous degeneration of valve
   L. Infective endocarditis
   M. After prosthetic valve surgery
   N. Associated with aortic stenosis
II. Acute aortic regurgitation
   A. Rheumatic fever
   B. Infective endocarditis
   C. Congenital (rupture of sinus of Valsalva)
   D. Acute aortic dissection
   E. After prosthetic valve surgery
   F. Trauma

*Please note that certain disorders are capable of producing acute and chronic aortic regurgitation.

SLE; Systemic lupus erythematosus.

From Hurst JW et al (eds): *The heart,* ed 8, New York, 1994, McGraw-Hill, p. 1467.

I-9   CAUSES OF TRICUSPID REGURGITATION
  I. Rheumatic heart disease
  II. Endocarditis
  III. Myocardial infarction (with or without papillary muscle dysfunction)
  IV. Trauma
  V. Pulmonary hypertension
  VI. Ebstein's anomaly
  VII. Endocardial pacemaker wire
  VIII. Pulmonary artery catheter (Swan-Ganz)
  IX. Carcinoid
  X. Rheumatoid arthritis
  XI. Radiation
  XII. Floppy (prolapse)

I-10   CLASSIFICATION OF ATRIAL SEPTAL DEFECTS
  I. Patent foramen ovale
  II. Persistent ostium secundum defect (fossa ovalis defect)
  III. Sinus venosus defect (proximal defect)
  IV. Endocardial cushion defect (complete and partial atrioventricular canal)
      A. Ostium primum defect (incomplete persistent common atrioventricular canal)
      B. Complete persistent common atrioventricular canal

I-11   CAUSES OF ATRIAL FLUTTER AND ATRIAL FIBRILLATION
  I. Valvular heart disease (mitral or tricuspid stenosis or regurgitation)
  II. Ischemic heart disease
  III. Hypertensive heart disease
  IV. Cardiomyopathy (dilated or hypertrophic)
  V. Congenital heart disease (atrial septal defect)
  VI. Pericarditis
  VII. Mitral valve prolapse
  VIII. Sick sinus syndrome
  IX. Pulmonary embolism
  X. Thyrotoxicosis
  XI. Hypoxemia of any etiology
  XII. Alcohol ingestion
  XIII. Atrial infarction
  XIV. After CABG

CABG, **Coronary artery bypass surgery.**

From Walsh K, Ezri M, Denes P: *Med Clin North Am* 70(4): 794, July, 1986.

I-12   COMPLICATIONS OF MITRAL STENOSIS

    I. Unrelated to severity of stenosis
        A. Atrial fibrillation
        B. Infective endocarditis
        C. Embolism
    II. Related to severity of stenosis
        A. Pulmonary edema
        B. Hemoptysis
        C. Dyspnea on exertion
        D. Pulmonary hypertension
        E. Right ventricular failure
    III. Chest x-ray findings in mitral stenosis
        A. Enlargement of left atrium
        B. Enlargement of right ventricle
        C. Kerley B lines
        D. Enlargement of the pulmonary artery
        E. Cephalization of the pulmonary vasculature
        F. Calcification in the area of the mitral valve

I-13   RISK FACTORS FOR ATHEROSCLEROTIC HEART DISEASE

    I. Hypercholesterolemia
        A. Low LDL
        B. High LDL
        C. High lipoprotein a Lp (a)
    II. Hypertension
    III. Tobacco use
    IV. Diabetes mellitus (abnormal glucose tolerance)
    V. Family history of atherosclerosis (MI, stroke, peripheral vascular disease)
    VI. Obesity
    VII. Sedentary living
    VIII. Type A personality
    IX. Oral contraceptive use
    X. Chronic obstructive lung disease
    XI. Chronic renal failure
    XII. Hypertriglyceridemia (type IV)
    XIII. Alcohol (greater than 3 oz distilled liquor or equivalent/day)
    XIV. Male (or postmenopausal female)
    XV. Immunosuppressive posttransplant
    XVI. Elevated fibrinogen
    XVII. Syndrome X (hypertriglyceridemia, hypertension, insulin resistance, centripetal obesity).
    XVIII. Hyperhomocystinemia

From Farmer JA, Gotto AM. In Braunwald E et al: *Heart disease: A textbook of cardiovascular medicine,* ed 4, Philadelphia, 1992, WB Saunders, pp 1125-1155.

I-14 PURPOSES OF ECG EXERCISE TESTS

ECG exercise tests may be performed for the following reasons:

I. Screening an asymptomatic population
   A. For prognostic evaluation, e.g., in general epidemiology surveys or of insurance applicants
   B. For investigations of groups at high risk for coronary disease, e.g., hyperlipidemic patients
   C. For study of workers in critical positions, e.g., commercial aircraft pilots, military pilots

II. For diagnostic evaluation of patients with chest pain not typical of angina pectoris

III. For evaluating the degree of ischemia in patients with known angina or previous infarction—with regard to prognosis, treatment, permitted exercise level

IV. For evaluating therapeutic procedures in patients with angina, e.g., coronary artery bypass grafting or trial of new drugs

V. For evaluating severity of other lesions, e.g., aortic stenosis in children, mitral stenosis (there is a general reluctance to exercise adults with aortic stenosis for fear of provoking ventricular dysrhythmias)

VI. For evaluating work capacity, e.g., after cardiac infarction.

VII. To evaluate entry into or the results of rehabilitation or exercise training programs.

VIII. To evaluate patients suspected of AV block or sinus node dysfunction.

I-15 MYOCARDIAL INFARCTION: CLINICAL AND HEMODYNAMIC SUBSETS

I. Class I
   A. Clinical: No evidence of heart failure
   B. Hemodynamic: PCWP = NML; CI > 2.2
   C. Prognosis: In hospital mortality 5%-7%*

II. Class II
   A. Clinical: Tachycardia, bibasilar rales to scapula tip and/or S_3 gallop
   B. Hemodynamic: PCWP > 18 mm Hg; CI > 2.2
   C. Prognosis: In hospital mortality 10%-15%*

III. Class III
   A. Clinical: Tachycardia, rales above tip of scapula, S_3 gallop or frank pulmonary edema
   B. Hemodynamic: PCWP ≤ 18; CI < 2.2
   C. Prognosis: In hospital mortality 25%-50%*

IV. Class IV (cardiogenic shock)
   A. Clinical: Hypotension, cool clammy extremities, mental confusion, decreased urine output
   B. Hemodynamic: PCWP > 18; CI < 2.2
   C. Prognosis: In hospital mortality 80%-90%*

*Current mortality may be lower (i.e., thrombolytics and angioplasty).

PCWP, Pulmonary capillary wedge pressure (mm Hg); *CI,* cardiac index (L/min/M^2).

From Killip III T, Kimball JT: Treatment of myocardial infarction in a coronary care unit, *Am J Cardiol* 20:457, 1967; Forrester J, Waters D: Hospital treatment of congestive heart failure: Management according to hemodynamic profile, *Am J Med* 65:73, 1978.

I-16   NONATHEROSCLEROTIC CAUSES OF MYOCARDIAL INFARCTION

I. Emboli to coronary arteries
  A. Thrombi from left ventricle (AMI, cardiomyopathy)
  B. Thrombi from left atrium (mitral stenosis)
  C. Thrombi from prosthetic valves
  D. Thrombi from catheters during angiography
  E. Air emboli (coronary angiography, cardiopulmonary bypass)
  F. Infectious and marantic endocarditis
  G. Atrial myxoma
II. Mechanical obstruction
  A. Chest trauma (contusion, laceration)
  B. Dissection of the aorta
  C. Dissection of coronary arteries (postpartum, post-PTCA, post-coronary angiography)
III. Increased vasomotor tone
  A. Variant angina
  B. Raynaud's disease
  C. Nitroglycerin withdrawal
IV. Arteritis
  A. Collagen vascular disease (PAN, SLE, RA, AS)
  B. Takayasu's disease
  C. Mucocutaneous lymph node (Kawasaki's) syndrome
  D. Luetic aortitis
V. Miscellaneous
  A. Anomalous origin and/or course of coronary arteries
  B. Hematologic disorders (DIC, PV)
  C. Aortic stenosis
  D. Hypertrophic cardiomyopathy
  E. Prolonged hypotension
  F. Cocaine

AMI, Anterior myocardial infarction; *PTCA,* percutaneous transcoronary angioplasty; *PAN,* polyarteritis nodosa; *AS,* ankylosing spondylitis; *PV,* Polycythemia vera.

From Cheitlin M, McAllister HA, Castro CM: Myocardial infarction without atherosclerosis, *JAMA* 231:951-955, 1975; Codini MA. In Bone RC et al (ed): *Med Clin North Am* 70(4): 771, 1986.

I-17   PROGNOSTIC DETERMINANTS IN ISCHEMIC HEART DISEASE

I. Objective severity of ischemia
   A. Treadmill
      1. Duration of exercise (failure to achieve 3 METS)
      2. Degree of ST depression/elevation during/postexercise
      3. Abnormal blood pressure response to exercise
      4. Exercise-induced ventricular ectopy
      5. Reversible ischemia with exercise by isotope
   B. Inability to perform exercise testing
II. Degree of left ventricular dysfunction
III. Recurrent ischemic events
   A. Myocardial infarction
   B. Unstable angina
   C. Cardiac sudden death
   D. Silent ischemia
   E. Postinfarction angina
IV. Extent of coronary atherosclerosis
V. Others
   A. History of hypertension
   B. History of congestive heart failure
   C. Cardiomegaly on chest x-ray
   D. ECG abnormalities
      1. Ventricular dysrhythmias
      2. Conduction defects
      3. Abnormal signal averaged ECG
      4. Inducible sustained monomorphic ventricular tachycardia during electrophysiologic testing
   E. Tobacco use
   F. Diabetes mellitus
   G. Age > 70
   H. Female sex
   I. Anterior myocardial infarction

From Pasternak RC, Braunwald E, Sobel BE. In Braunwald E: *Heart disease: A textbook of cardiovascular medicine,* ed 4, Philadelphia, 1992, WB Saunders, p. 1267.

I-18   PSEUDOINFARCTION ECG PATTERNS

   I. Myocardial replacement
      A. Tumor
      B. Abscess
      C. Amyloid disease
      D. Pseudohypertrophic muscular dystrophy
      E. Sarcoid involving the heart
      F. Friedreich's ataxia
      G. Muscular dystrophy
   II. Nonmyocardial replacement
      A. Anatomic factors
         1. Emphysema
         2. Pneumothorax
      B. Inflammatory conditions
         1. Myocarditis
         2. Pericarditis
  III. Depolarization abnormalities
      A. IHSS
      B. WPW syndrome
      C. LBBB, LAFB
  IV. Right ventricular hypertrophy
      A. Cor pulmonale
      B. Mitral stenosis
   V. Left ventricular disease
      A. Left ventricular hypertrophy
      B. Congestive cardiomyopathy
      C. Left ventricular aneurysm
  VI. Dysrhythmias
      A. Ventricular tachycardia
      B. Electronic pacing of right ventricle
 VII. Congestive cardiomyopathy
VIII. Hyperkalemia
  IX. Intracranial hemorrhage
   X. Trauma
  XI. Early repolarization pattern
 XII. Hypothermia

IHSS, **Idiopathic hypertrophic subaortic stenosis;** *WPW,* **Wolff-Parkinson-White;** *LBBB,* **left bundle branch block;** *LAFB,* **left anterior fascicular block.**

From Fisch C. In Braunwald E: *Heart disease: A textbook of cardiovascular medicine,* ed 4, Philadelphia, 1992, WB Saunders, pp. 116-153.

I-19 CAUSES OF SUDDEN, NONTRAUMATIC DEATH

I. Cardiac
   A. Atherosclerotic coronary artery disease
   B. Stokes-Adams syndrome
   C. Valvular heart disease
      1. Aortic stenosis
      2. Mitral valve prolapse
   D. Myocarditis
   E. Acute pericardial tamponade
   F. Primary myocardial disease
   G. Congestive heart disease
   H. Prolonged Q-T interval syndrome
   I. Drug effects
      1. Hypokalemia and hyperkalemia
      2. Digitalis
      3. Quinidine and other type I antiarrhythmics
      4. Tricyclic antidepressants
      5. Cocaine
   J. Anomalous conduction pathways
      1. Wolff-Parkinson-White
      2. Lown-Ganong-Levin
   K. Conduction system disease

II. Pulmonary
   A. Cor pulmonale
      1. Acute
      2. Chronic
   B. Status asthmaticus
   C. Asphyxia
      1. Cafe coronary

III. Extracardiac
   A. Dissecting aortic aneurysm
   B. Exsanguinating hemorrhage
   C. Cerebrovascular accident

IV. Miscellaneous
   A. Sudden infant death syndrome
   B. Acute pancreatitis
   C. Unexplained

I-20   RISK FACTORS FOR ANTICOAGULATION

   I. Preexisting coagulation defect
   II. Ulcerative lesion in the GI tract (peptic ulcer, ulcerative colitis)
   III. Salicylate therapy
   IV. Old age >75 years
   V. Poor patient compliance
   VI. Pregnancy
   VII. Infective endocarditis
   VIII. Liver disease
   IX. Advanced retinopathy
   X. Malignant hypertension
   XI. Recent CVA or intracranial process
   XII. Unsteady gait

I-21 ETIOLOGIC CLASSIFICATION OF CARDIOMYOPATHIES

I. Primary myocardial involvement
  A. Idiopathic (D,R,H)
  B. Familial (D,H)
  C. Eosinophilic endomyocardial disease (R)
  D. Endomyocardial fibrosis (R)
II. Secondary myocardial involvement
  A. Infective (D)
    1. Viral myocarditis
    2. Bacterial myocarditis
    3. Fungal myocarditis
    4. Protozoal myocarditis
    5. Metazoal myocarditis
    6. Spirochetal
    7. Rickettsial
  B. Metabolic (D)
  C. Familial storage disease (D,R)
    1. Glycogen storage disease
    2. Mucopolysaccharidoses
  D. Deficiency (D)
    1. Electrolytes
    2. Nutritional
  E. Connective tissue disorders (D)
    1. SLE
    2. Polyarteritis nodosa
    3. Rheumatoid arthritis
    4. Scleroderma
    5. Dermatomyositis

Continued

I-21   ETIOLOGIC CLASSIFICATION
OF CARDIOMYOPATHIES—*cont'd*

F. Infiltrations and granulomas (R,D)
1. Amyloidosis
2. Sarcoidosis
3. Malignancy
4. Hemochromatosis
G. Neuromuscular (D)
1. Muscular dystrophy
2. Myotonic dystrophy
3. Friedreich's ataxia (H,D)
4. Refsum's disease
H. Sensitivity and toxic reactions (D)
1. Alcohol
2. Radiation
3. Drugs (daunorubicin)
I. Peripartum heart disease (D)
J. Endocardial fibroelastosis (R)
K. Obesity (D)

Note: **The principal clinical manifestation(s) of each etiologic grouping is denoted by** *D* **(dilated),** *R* **(restrictive), or** *H* **(hypertrophic cardiomyopathy).**

From the WHO/ISFC task force report on the definition and classification of cardiomyopathies, 1980.

From Isselbacher KJ et al (eds): *Harrison's principles of internal medicine,* ed 13, New York City, 1994, McGraw-Hill, p. 1089.

I-22   CONGESTIVE HEART FAILURE: PRECIPITATING CAUSES

   I. Pulmonary embolism
  II. Myocardial infarction
 III. Dysrhythmias
  IV. Increasingly severe hypertension
   V. Noncompliance with medications
      A. Digitalis
      B. Diuretics
      C. Vasodilators
  VI. Excess dietary sodium
 VII. Excess amounts of intravenous fluids
VIII. Drugs
      A. Propranolol and other beta blockers
      B. Cardiotoxic drugs
         1. Daunorubicin
      C. NSAIDs
      D. Antidysrhythmics (disopyramide)
      E. Corticosteroids
      F. Androgens and estrogens
      G. Tricycle psychotropic drugs (e.g., nortriptyline)
      H. Cocaine
  IX. Pregnancy
   X. High output states with increased metabolic demands
      A. Fever
      B. Hyperthyroidism
      C. Anemia
      D. AV fistula
      E. Infections
      F. Paget's disease
      G. Thiamine deficiency
  XI. Rheumatic and other forms of myocarditis
 XII. Alcohol
XIII. Infective endocarditis
XIV. Hypothyroidism
 XV. Renal failure

I-23   REVERSIBLE CAUSES OF CONGESTIVE HEART FAILURE

   I. Anemia
   II. Hyperthyroidism/hypothyroidism
   III. Atrial myxoma
   IV. Arteriovenous fistula
   V. Surgically correctable valvular heart disease
   VI. Surgically correctable congenital heart disease
   VII. Cardiac dysrhythmias in an otherwise normal heart
   VIII. Thiamine deficiency
   IX. Alcohol
   X. Obesity
   XI. Paget's disease

I-24   POTENTIAL LIFE-THREATENING COMPLICATIONS OF ACUTE MYOCARDIAL INFARCTION

Ventricular dysrhythmias (ventricular tachycardia, ventricular fibrillation, or asystole)

Extremely rapid atrial dysrhythmias in association with extensive myocardial infarction (atrial flutter or atrial fibrillation)

Heart block (second- or third-degree)

Marked bradycardia

Loss of atrial contribution to cardiac contraction (atrioventricular junctional rhythm)

Infarction $\geq 40\%$ of left ventricle

Extensive right ventricular infarction

Acute and severe mitral regurgitation

Severe pulmonary edema

Rupture of the heart

Systemic and/or pulmonary emboli

Cardiogenic shock

Infarct extension

From Wyngaarden JB, Smith Jr LH (eds): *Cecil textbook of medicine*, Philadelphia, 1988, WB Saunders, p. 336.

I-25 TYPES OF HYPERTENSION

I. Systolic and diastolic hypertension
  A. Primary, essential, or idiopathic
  B. Secondary
    1. Renal
      a. Renal parenchymal disease
        (1) Acute glomerulonephritis
        (2) Chronic nephritis
        (3) Polycystic disease
        (4) Connective tissue diseases
        (5) Diabetic nephropathy
        (6) Hydronephrosis
      b. Renovascular
      c. Renin-producing tumors
      d. Renoprival
      e. Primary sodium retention (Liddle's syndrome, Gordon's syndrome)
    2. Endocrine
      a. Acromegaly
      b. Hypothyroidism
      c. Hypercalcemia
      d. Hyperthyroidism
      e. Adrenal
        (1) Cortical
          (a) Cushing's syndrome
          (b) Primary aldosteronism
          (c) Congenital adrenal hyperplasia
        (2) Medullary: pheochromocytoma
      f. Extra-adrenal chromaffin tumors
      g. Carcinoid
      h. Exogenous hormones
        (1) Estrogen
        (2) Glucocorticoid
        (3) Mineralocorticoids: licorice, carbenoxolone
        (4) Sympathomimetics
        (5) Tyramine-containing foods and MAO inhibitors

Continued

I-25 TYPES OF HYPERTENSION—*cont'd*

    3. Coarctation of the aorta
    4. Pregnancy-induced hypertension
    5. Neurologic disorders
       a. Increased intracranial pressure
         (1) Brain tumor
         (2) Encephalitis
         (3) Respiratory acidosis: lung or CNS disease
       b. Quadriplegia
       c. Acute porphyria
       d. Familial dysautonomia (Riley-Day)
       e. Lead poisoning
       f. Guillain-Barré syndrome
    6. Acute stress, including surgery
       a. Psychogenic hyperventilation
       b. Hypoglycemia
       c. Burns
       d. Pancreatitis
       e. Alcohol withdrawal
       f. Sickle cell crisis
       g. Postresuscitation
       h. Postoperative
    7. Increased intravascular volume
    8. Drugs and other substances
  II. Systolic hypertension
    A. Increased cardiac output
       1. Aortic valvular regurgitation
       2. AV fistula, patent ductus
       3. Thyrotoxicosis
       4. Paget's disease of bone
       5. Beriberi
       6. Hyperkinetic circulation
    B. Rigidity of aorta

From Kaplan NM. In Braunwald E: *Heart disease: A textbook of cardiovascular medicine,* ed 4, Philadelphia, 1992, WB Saunders, p. 820.

I-26 FACTORS INDICATING AN ADVERSE PROGNOSIS IN HYPERTENSION

   I. Black race
   II. Youth
   III. Male
   IV. Persistent diastolic pressure >115 mm Hg
   V. Smoking
   VI. Diabetes mellitus
   VII. Hypercholesterolemia
   VIII. Obesity
   IX. Evidence of end organ damage
      A. Cardiac
         1. Cardiac enlargement
         2. ECG changes of ischemic or left ventricular strain
         3. Myocardial infarction
         4. Congestive heart failure
      B. Eyes
         1. Retinal exudates and hemorrhages
         2. Papilledema
      C. Renal: impaired renal function
      D. Nervous system: cerebrovascular accident

From Williams GH et al. In Isselbacher KJ et al (eds): *Harrison's principles of internal medicine,* ed 13, McGraw Hill, 1994, New York, p. 1119.

I-27 ETIOLOGY OF SYNCOPE, WEAKNESS, AND FAINTNESS

   I. Circulatory (deficient quantity of blood to the brain)
      A. Inadequate vasoconstrictor mechanisms
         1. Vasovagal (vasodepression)
         2. Postural hypotension
         3. Primary autonomic insufficiency
         4. Sympathectomy (pharmacologic due to antihypertensive medications, such as Aldomet and hydralazine, or surgical)
         5. Diseases of central and peripheral nervous systems, including autonomic nerves
         6. Carotid sinus syncope (see also "Bradydysrhythmias")
         7. Hyperbradykininemia
      B. Hypovolemia
         1. Blood loss—gastrointestinal hemorrhage
         2. Addison's disease
      C. Mechanical reduction of venous return
         1. Valsalva maneuver
         2. Cough (posttussive)
         3. Micturition
         4. Atrial myxoma, ball valve thrombus

Continued

I-27   ETIOLOGY OF SYNCOPE, WEAKNESS, AND FAINTNESS—*cont'd*

D. Reduced cardiac output
   1. Obstruction to left ventricular outflow: Aortic stenosis, hypertrophic subaortic stenosis
   2. Obstruction to pulmonic flow: Pulmonic stenosis, primary pulmonary hypertension, pulmonary embolism
   3. Myocardial: Massive myocardial infarction with pump failure
   4. Pericardial: Cardiac tamponade
E. Dysrhythmias
   1. Bradydysrhythmias
      a. Atrioventricular (AV) block (second- and third-degree), with Stokes-Adams attacks
      b. Ventricular asystole
      c. Sinus bradycardia, sinoatrial block, sinus arrest
      d. Carotid sinus syncope (see also Inadequate Vasoconstrictor Mechanisms)
      e. Glossopharyngeal neuralgia (and other painful states)
   2. Tachydysrhythmias
      a. Episodic ventricular tachycardia with or without associated bradydysrhythmias
      b. Supraventricular tachycardia without AV block
II. Other causes of weakness and episodic disturbances of consciousness
A. Altered state of blood to the brain
   1. Hypoxia
   2. Anemia
   3. Diminished carbon dioxide due to hyperventilation (faintness common, syncope seldom occurs)
   4. Hypoglycemia (episodic weakness common, faintness occasional, syncope rare)
B. Cerebral
   1. Cerebrovascular disturbances (TIAs, etc)
      a. Extracranial vascular insufficiency (vertebral-basilar, carotid)
      b. Diffuse spasm of cerebral arterioles (hypertensive encephalopathy)
   2. Emotional disturbances, anxiety attacks, and hysterical seizures

From Ruskin J, Martin J. In Isselbacher KJ et al (eds): *Harrison's principles of internal medicine,* ed 13, New York, 1994, McGraw Hill, p. 91.

I-28   CLASSIFICATION OF PERICARDITIS

I. Clinical classification
   A. Acute pericarditis (6 weeks)
      1. Fibrinous
      2. Effusive (or bloody)
   B. Subacute pericarditis (6 weeks to 6 months)
      1. Constrictive
      2. Effusive-constrictive
   C. Chronic pericarditis (>6 months)
      1. Constructive
      2. Effusive
      3. Adhesive (nonconstrictive)
II. Etiologic classification
   A. Infectious pericarditis
      1. Viral
      2. Pyogenic
      3. Tuberculous
      4. Mycotic
      5. Other infections (syphilitic, parasitic)
   B. Noninfectious pericarditis
      1. Acute myocardial infarction
      2. Uremia
      3. Neoplasia
         a. Primary tumors (benign or malignant)
         b. Tumors metastatic to pericardium
      4. Myxedema
      5. Cholesterol
      6. Chylopericardium
      7. Trauma
         a. Penetrating chest wall
         b. Nonpenetrating
      8. Aortic aneurysm (with leakage into pericardial sac)
      9. Postirradiation
      10. Associated with atrial septal defect
      11. Associated with severe chronic anemia
      12. Infectious mononucleosis
      13. Familial Mediterranean fever
      14. Familial pericarditis
         a. Mulibrey nanism*
      15. Sarcoidosis
      16. Acute idiopathic

Continued

I-28   CLASSIFICATION OF PERICARDITIS—*cont'd*

C. Pericarditis presumably related to hypersensitivity of autoimmunity
1. Rheumatic fever
2. Collagen vascular disease
   a. SLE
   b. Rheumatoid arthritis
   c. Scleroderma
3. Drug-induced
   a. Procainamide
   b. Hydralazine
   c. Other
4. Postcardiac injury
   a. Postmyocardial infarction (Dressler's syndrome)
   b. Postpericardiotomy

*An autosomal recessive syndrome, characterized by growth failure, muscle hypotonia, hepatomegaly, ocular changes, enlarged cerebral ventricles, mental retardation, and chronic constrictive pericarditis.

From Braunwald E. In Isselbacher KJ et al (eds): *Harrison's principles of internal medicine*, ed 13, New York, 1994, McGraw Hill, p. 1095.

I-29   ETIOLOGY OF CHRONIC CONSTRICTIVE PERICARDITIS

I. Unknown
II. After idiopathic pericarditis
III. Specific infection
   A. Bacterial
   B. Tuberculosis (50% to 65% of treated pericarditis)
   C. Fungal disease (rare): histoplasmosis, coccidioidomycosis
   D. Viral disease, especially Coxsackie B_3
   E. Parasitic disease: amebiasis, echinococcosis
IV. Connective tissue disease: rheumatoid arthritis, SLE
V. Neoplastic disease
   A. Primary mesothelioma
   B. Secondary lymphoma, bronchogenic carcinoma, breast
VI. Trauma
   A. Blunt or penetrating
   B. Surgical (rare)
VII. Radiation therapy
VIII. Uremic
IX. Hereditary (Mulibrey nanism—Finland)

I-30 CLINICAL FEATURES OF CONSTRICTIVE PERICARDITIS (137 CASES)

I. Symptoms
   A. Effort dyspnea—89.8%
   B. Chest pain—24%*
   C. RUQ or epigastric pain—10.9%
   D. Effort syncope—4
   E. Orthopnea, paroxysmal nocturnal dyspnea—3
II. Physical findings
   A. Atrial fibrillation—27%
   B. Cervical veins engorged; venous pressure 15-44 cm H_2O
   C. Liver enlarged—134 cases
   D. Ascites—77.4%
   E. Peripheral edema—61%
   F. Pleural effusion—47%
   G. Paradoxical pulse—29%
   H. Early diastolic heart sound—20 cases

*Most studies do not report so high a prevalence of chest pain.
From Hirschmann JV: Am Heart J 96:111, 1978; Wychulis et al: *J Thorac Cardiovasc Surg* 62:608, 1971.

I-31   ETIOLOGY OF PERICARDIAL EFFUSION

I. Serous
- A. Congestive heart failure
- B. Hypoalbuminemia
- C. Irradiation
- D. Viral pericarditis
- E. Tuberculous pericarditis
- F. Bacterial pericarditis
- G. Dressler's syndrome
- H. Chemotherapeutic agents
- I. Myxedema

II. Blood (hematocrit >10%)
- A. Iatrogenic
  1. Cardiac operation
  2. Cardiac catheterization
  3. Trauma (penetrating and nonpenetrating)
  4. Anticoagulant agents
  5. Chemotherapeutic agents
- B. Neoplasm
- C. Trauma
- D. Acute myocardial infarction
- E. Cardiac rupture
- F. Rupture of ascending aorta or major pulmonary artery
- G. Coagulopathy
- H. Uremia

III. Lymph or chyle
- A. Neoplasm
- B. Iatrogenic
  1. Cardiothoracic surgery
- C. Congenital
- D. Idiopathic ("primary chylopericardium")
- E. Nonneoplastic obstruction of thoracic duct

From Shabetai R. In Plum F, Bennett JC (eds): *Cecil textbook of medicine,* ed 20, *Philadelphia, 1996, WB Saunders, p. 337.*

I-32 COMMON ETIOLOGIES OF CARDIAC TAMPONADE

	1980 (%)	1988 (%)
DISORDER		
Malignant disease	32	58
Idiopathic pericarditis	14	14
Uremia	9	14
Acute cardiac infarction (receiving heparin)	9	—
Diagnostic procedures with cardiac perforation	7.5	—
Bacterial	7.5	5
Tuberculosis	5	1
Radiation	4	—
Myxedema	4	—
Dissecting aortic aneurysm	4	—
Postpericardiotomy syndrome	2	—
SLE	2	2
Cardiomyopathy (receiving anticoagulants)	2	6

From Lorell BH, Braunwald E. In Braunwald E et al (eds): *Heart disease: A textbook of cardiovascular medicine,* ed 4, Philadelphia, 1992, WB Saunders, p. 1476.

I-33   PREDISPOSING FACTORS TO CHRONIC PULMONARY HYPERTENSION AND COR PULMONALE

I. Hypoxic vasoconstriction
   A. Chronic bronchitis and emphysema, cystic fibrosis
   B. Chronic hypoventilation
      1. Obesity
      2. Sleep apnea
      3. Neuromuscular disease
      4. Chest wall dysfunction
      5. Primary or idiopathic alveolar hypoventilation ("Ondine's curse")
   C. High-altitude dwelling and chronic mountain sickness
II. Occlusion of the pulmonary vascular bed
   A. Pulmonary thromboembolism, parasitic ova, tumor emboli
   B. Primary pulmonary hypertension
   C. Pulmonary venoocclusive disease
   D. Fibrosing mediastinitis, mediastinal tumor
   E. Pulmonary angiitis from systemic disease
      1. Collagen vascular diseases
      2. Drug-induced lung disease
      3. Necrotizing and granulomatous arteritis
III. Parenchymal disease with loss of vascular surface area
   A. Bullous emphysema, α_1 antitrypsin deficiency
   B. Diffuse bronchiectasis, cystic fibrosis
   C. Diffuse interstitial disease
      1. Pneumoconioses
      2. Sarcoid, idiopathic pulmonary fibrosis, histiocytosis X
      3. Tuberculosis, chronic fungal infection
      4. ARDS
      5. Collagen vascular disease (immune lung disease)
      6. Hypersensitivity pneumonitis
IV. Cardiac disease
   A. Acquired disorders of the left side of the heart causing pulmonary venous hypertension
      1. Left ventricular failure
      2. Mitral valve disease
      3. Left atrial myxoma
      4. Decrease in left ventricular compliance
   B. Congenital heart disease
      1. Pre-tricuspid
      2. Post-tricuspid

From Hurst JW et al (eds): *The heart,* ed 7, New York, 1990, McGraw Hill, p. 1220.

I-34   PULMONARY VALVULAR INSUFFICIENCY

I. Congenital
   A. With tetralogy of Fallot
   B. With Eisenmenger's syndrome
   C. With Marfan's syndrome
   D. Isolated
   E. With patent ductus arteriosus
   F. With idiopathic dilation of the pulmonary artery

II. Acquired as a result of other congenital heart disease.
   A. After operation on the stenotic pulmonary valve
   B. With pulmonary hypertension related to patent ductus arteriosus, atrial septal defect, or ventricular septal defect

III. As a result of acquired heart disease
   A. With idiopathic or thromboembolic pulmonary hypertension
   B. With mitral stenosis
   C. With bacterial endocarditis
   D. With rheumatic fever
   E. With syphilis
   F. With carcinoid syndrome
   G. With aneurysm of the pulmonary artery (often syphilitic)
   H. With pulmonary hypertension and chronic lung disease

I-35 FACTORS PREDISPOSING TO THROMBOEMBOLISM

I. Heart disease, especially the following:
   A. Myocardial infarction
   B. Atrial fibrillation
   C. Cardiomyopathy
   D. Congestive heart failure
II. Postoperative state, especially operations on abdomen or pelvis, splenectomy, and orthopedic procedures on lower extremities
III. Pregnancy and parturition
IV. Neoplastic disease
V. Polycythemia
VI. Prolonged immobilization
VII. Hemorrhage
VIII. Fractures, especially of the hip
IX. Obesity
X. Varicose veins
XI. Prior history of thromboembolic disease
XII. Certain drugs: oral contraceptives, estrogens
XIII. After cerebrovascular accidents
XIV. Abnormal blood flow
XV. Myeloproliferative disorders with thrombocytosis
XVI. Antithrombin III deficiency
XVII. Protein C deficiency, protein S deficiency
XVIII. Abnormal fibrinolysis
XIX. Factor V Leiden mutation
XX. Antiphospholipid antibody syndrome

I-36 DIGITALIS INTOXICATION

I. Patients with increased risk of digitalis intoxication
   A. Renal insufficiency or failure
   B. Malabsorption
   C. Elderly patients
   D. Obese patients
   E. Electrolyte imbalance (decreased K+, increased CA++, decreased Mg++)
   F. Liver disease (digitoxin only)
   G. Thyroid disease (hypothyroidism)
   H. Pulmonary disease
   I. Drugs (quinidine, verapamil, diltiazem, amiodarone, and procainamide)
II. Diagnosis of digitalis intoxication
   *A. Symptoms: diarrhea, anorexia, nausea, emesis, visual disturbances
   *B. Dysrhythmias
   *C. Digitalis dose excessive for body weight
      1. Usual maintenance dose of digoxin is 3 μg/kg
   *D. Digitalis dose excessive in the presence of impaired renal function
   *E. Increased serum digitalis glycoside levels
   *F. Improvement in items A, B, and E after discontinuation of and/or readjustment in glycoside dosage

*These findings are not always present.

1-37   ASSESSMENT OF CARDIOVASCULAR RISK IN PATIENTS BEING CONSIDERED FOR SURGERY

Risk factor present	Points
I. History	
A. Age > 70	5
B. Myocardial infarction previous 6 mo.	10
II. Physical examination	
A. Aortic stenosis	3
B. Signs of congestive heart failure, S_3 gallop, jugular venous distention	11
III. Cardiac rhythm	
A. Premature ventricular contractions	7
B. Rhythm other than normal sinus	7
IV. Miscellaneous	
A. Emergent procedure	4
B. Intrathoracic/intraabdominal procedure	3
C. ↑ Bun, ↓ serum K+, ↓ arterial po_2	3
Total possible points	53
V. Assessment of risk	
0 to 5 points (minimal)	Grade I
6 to 12 points (minimal to moderate)	Grade II
13 to 25 points (moderate to severe)	Grade III
>26 points (prohibitive)	Grade IV

From Goldman L: *New Engl J Med* 297:845, 1977.

I-38 CLASSIFICATION OF ANTIDYSRHYTHMIC DRUGS ACCORDING TO THEIR MECHANISM OF ACTION

Class action	Drugs
I. Fast sodium channel blockade	
A. Reduce $V_{max,}$ prolong action potential duration	Quinidine, procainamide, disopyramide
B. Do not change $V_{max,}$ shorten action potential duration	Tocainide, mexiletine, phenytoin, lidocaine, probably moricizine
C. Reduce $V_{max,}$ primarily slow conduction; can prolong refractoriness	Encainide, propafenone
II. Beta-adrenergic blockade	Esmolol, propranolol, timolol, metaprolol, sotalol, others
III. Block potassium channels, prolong repolarization	Sotalol, amiodarone, bretylium, *N*-acetyl-procainamide
IV. Calcium channel blockade	Verapamil, diltiazem, nifedipine, others

From Zipes DP. In Braunwald E et al: *Heart disease: A textbook of cardiovascular medicine,* Philadelphia, 1992, WB Saunders, p. 628.

I-39   DEFINITE INDICATIONS FOR IMPLANTED PACEMAKER

I. Complete heart block, permanent or intermittent, with any one of the following complications:
   A. Symptomatic bradycardia
   B. Congestive heart failure
   C. Conditions that require treatment with drugs that suppress ventricular escape rhythms
   D. Asystole $\geq$3 seconds or ventricular rate <40 per minute.
   E. Mental confusion that clears with pacing

II. Patients with complete heart block or advanced second-degree AV block that persists after myocardial infarction

III. Chronic bifascicular or trifascicular block with intermittent complete heart block or type II second-degree AV block associated with symptomatic bradycardia.

IV. Sinus node dysfunction with documented symptomatic bradycardia

V. Hypersensitive carotid sinus syndrome with recurrent syncope and asystole >3 seconds provoked by minimal carotid sinus pressure

VI. Symptomatic supraventricular tachycardia that does not respond to medical treatment.

From Barold SS, Zipes DP. In Braunwald E: *Heart disease: A textbook of cardiovascular medicine,* ed 4, Philadelphia, 1992, WB Saunders, p. 728.

I-40 INDICATIONS FOR CLINICAL ELECTROPHYSIOLOGICAL STUDIES— ENDOCARDIAL ELECTRICAL STIMULATION

I. To evaluate mechanism, site, and extent of dysrhythmia and/or conduction defect.
   A. Sick sinus syndrome
   B. Pre-excitation syndrome
   C. Supraventricular tachycardia
   D. Distinguish between supraventricular dysrhythmias with aberration and ventricular dysrhythmia
   E. Type I AV block with bundle branch block
   F. Type II AV block with normal QRS
   G. Bifascicular block occurring in acute myocardial infarction

II. To search for a cause for syncope
   A. Evaluate sinus node function
   B. Evaluate AV node function
   C. Evaluate function of His-Purkinje system
   D. Evaluate functional characteristics of anomalous AV connections
   E. Provoke dysrhythmias
      1. Supraventricular tachycardia
      2. Atrial flutter or fibrillation
      3. Ventricular tachycardia

III. To evaluate therapy
   A. Drug therapy
      1. Prevent inducible dysrhythmias
      2. Measure conduction and refractoriness in anomalous AV connections
      3. Evaluate adverse effects
         a. Sinus node function
         b. AV node function
         c. His-Purkinje system
         d. Effect on device function
   B. Catheter ablation or surgical therapy
      1. Preoperative endocardial catheter mapping
         a. Location of anomalous AV connections
         b. Location of VT circuit
         c. Need for concomitant pacemaker implantation
      2. Postoperative evaluation
         a. Presence of anomalous AV connections
         b. Dysrhythmia inducible

Continued

I-40   INDICATIONS FOR CLINICAL ELECTROPHYSIOLOGICAL STUDIES— ENDOCARDIAL ELECTRICAL STIMULATION—*cont'd*

    C. AICD therapy

        1. Preoperative evaluation

            a. Determine that VT or VF is inducible

            b. Determine that VT or VF is drug resistant

            c. Determine need for concomitant pacemaker implantation

        2. Intraoperative evaluation

            a. Determine quality of right or left ventricular sensing electrograms

            b. Determine quality of patch electrograms for the probability density function.

            c. Determine defibrillation thresholds

            d. Induce clinical dysrhythmia to test sensing and termination of ventricular dysrhythmias by the AICD

        3. Postoperative evaluation

            a. Induce VT or VF to test the performance of the AICD

            b. Acquaint the patient with the symptoms during AICD discharge

    D. Pacemaker therapy

        1. Evaluate condition for suitability for pacemaker therapy

            a. Supraventricular tachycardia-reciprocation in the AV node

            b. Supraventricular tachycardia-reciprocation in anomalous AV connections

        2. Determine the information needed to select pacemaker type and parameters

  IV. To apply ablation therapy

    A. Posterior septal anomalous AV connections

    B. AV node

    C. Ventricular tachycardia

AICD, Automatic implantable cardioverter defibrillator; *VT,* ventricular tachycardia; *VF,* ventricular fibrillation.

From Bigger JT. In Plum F, Bennett JC (eds): *Cecil textbook of medicine,* ed 20, Philadelphia, 1996, WB Saunders, p. 236.

I-41 NBG PACEMAKER CODE

		Code positions*		
I† Chamber paced	II† Chamber paced	III Response to sensing	IV Programmable functions; rate-modulation	V Antitachyarrhythmia functions
C V-ventricle	V-ventricle	T-triggers	P-programmable rate or output	P-anti-pacing tachydysrhythmia
O A-atrium	A-atrium	I-inhibits pacing	M-multiprogram ability of rate, sensitivity, etc.	S-shock
D D-double	D-double	D-triggers and inhibits pacing		D-dual (P + S)
E O-none	O-none	O-none		O-none
L			C-communicating functions (telemetry)	
E			R-rare modulation	
T			O-none	
T				
E				
R				
S				

*Positions I-III are used exclusively for antibradydysrhythmia pacing.
†Manufacturers often use "S" for single-chamber (A or V).
From Mond SJ, Sloman J. In Hurst JW et al: *The heart*, ed 8, New York, 1994, McGraw Hill, p. 826.

I-42   CAUSES OF SHOCK AND INITIATING MECHANISMS

I. Hypovolemic shock
  A. Hemorrhagic (e.g., trauma, gastrointestinal hemorrhage)
  B. Hypovolemic, nonhemorrhagic
    1. External fluid loss (e.g., vomiting diarrhea, polyuria, burns)
    2. Internal extravascular sequestration (e.g., peritonitis, pancreatitis)
II. Cardiogenic shock
  A. Acute myocardial infarction
    1. Loss of critical muscle mass (e.g., large anterior wall infarction)
    2. Acute mechanical lesion (e.g., ventricular septal rupture, mitral insufficiency)
    3. Acute right ventricular infarction
    4. Left ventricular free wall rupture
    5. Left ventricular aneurysm
  B. Valvular heart disease
    1. Critical valvular stenosis (e.g., aortic or mitral stenosis)
    2. Severe valvular insufficiency (e.g., acute aortic or mitral insufficiency)
  C. Nonvalvular obstructive cardiac lesions
    1. Atrial myxoma or ball-valve thrombus
    2. Cardiac tamponade
    3. Restrictive cardiomyopathy (e.g., amyloid)
    4. Constrictive pericardial disorder
  D. Nonischemic myopathic processes
    1. Fulminant myocarditis
    2. Physiologic depressants (e.g., acidosis, hypoxia)
    3. Pharmacologic depressants (e.g., calcium channel blockers)
    4. Pathophysiologic depressants (e.g., myocardial depressant factor)
  E. Dysrhythmias
    1. Severe bradydysrhythmias (e.g., high-degree AV block)
    2. Tachydysrhythmias
      a. Ventricular (e.g., ventricular tachycardia)
      b. Supraventricular (e.g., atrial fibrillation or flutter with rapid ventricular response)
III. Vascular obstructive shock
  A. Massive pulmonary embolism
  B. Tension pneumothorax
  C. Excessive positive-pressure ventilation
  D. Aortic dissection

Continued

I-42   CAUSES OF SHOCK AND INITIATING MECHANISMS—*cont'd*

   IV. Distributive shock and miscellaneous
      A. Sepsis
      B. Anaphylaxis
      C. Massive tissue injury (e.g., crush)
      D. Prolonged ischemia/hypoxia
      E. Neurogenic shock
      F. Endocrine disorders
         1. Addisonian crisis
         2. Profound hypothyroidism
      G. Drug or toxin induced

From Ferguson DW. In Wyngaarden JB et al (eds): *Cecil textbook of medicine*, ed 19, Philadelphia, 1992, WB Saunders, p.216.

I-43   CONTRAINDICATIONS OF THROMBOLYTIC THERAPY

   I. Absolute contraindications
      A. Aortic dissection
      B. Acute pericarditis
      C. Active bleeding
      D. Previous cerebral hemorrhage, cerebral neoplasm, intracranial vascular disease (aneurysm, AVM)
   II. Relative contraindications*
      A. Potential bleeding focus
         1. Within the past 6 months:
            GI or genitourinary hemorrhage or stroke
         2. Within the past 2-4 weeks:
            Major surgery, organ biopsy, puncture of noncompressible vessel, chest compression, major trauma, minor head trauma
         3. Diabetic proliferative retinopathy
         4. Severe, uncontrolled hypertension
            (systolic BP > 200 mm Hg, diastolic BP > 120 mm Hg)
      B. History of bleeding diathesis, hepatic dysfunction, cancer
      C. Pregnancy

*Physician must attempt to estimate for given patient benefit and risk of thrombolytic therapy.

From Cairns JA et al: *Chest* 108(4):417S, 1995.

I-44 BACTERIAL ENDOCARDITIS PROPHYLAXIS*

I. Cardiac conditions
  A. Endocarditis prophylaxis recommended
    1. Prosthetic cardiac valves, including bioprosthetic and homograft valves
    2. Previous bacterial endocarditis, even in the absence of heart disease
    3. Most congenital cardiac malformations
    4. Rheumatic and other acquired valvular dysfunction, even after valvular surgery
    5. Hypertrophic cardiomyopathy
    6. Mitral valve prolapse with valvular regurgitation
  B. Endocarditis prophylaxis not recommended
    1. Isolated secundum atrial septal defect
    2. Surgical repair without residua beyond 6 mo of secundum atrial septal defect, ventricular septal defect, or patent ductus arteriosus
    3. Previous coronary artery bypass graft surgery
    4. Mitral valve prolapse without valvular regurgitation†
    5. Physiologic, functional, or innocent heart murmurs
    6. Previous Kawasaki disease without valvular dysfunction
    7. Previous rheumatic fever without valvular dysfunction
    8. Cardiac pacemakers and implanted defibrillators
II. Dental or surgical procedures
  A. Endocarditis prophylaxis recommended
    1. Dental procedures known to induce gingival or mucosal bleeding, including professional cleaning
    2. Tonsillectomy and/or adenoidectomy
    3. Surgical operations that involve intestinal or respiratory mucosa
    4. Bronchoscopy with a rigid bronchoscope
    5. Sclerotherapy for esophageal varices
    6. Esophageal dilatation
    7. Gallbladder surgery
    8. Cystoscopy
    9. Urethral dilatation
    10. Urethral catheterization if urinary tract infection is present**
    11. Urinary tract surgery if urinary tract infection is present**
    12. Prostatic surgery
    13. Incision and drainage of infected tissue**
    14. Vaginal hysterectomy
    15. Vaginal delivery in the presence of infection**
  B. Endocarditis prophylaxis not recommended‡
    1. Dental procedures not likely to induce gingival bleeding, such as simple adjustment of orthodontic appliances or fillings above the gum line
    2. Injection of local intraoral anesthetic (except intraligamentary injections)

Continued

I-44 BACTERIAL ENDOCARDITIS PROPHYLAXIS—*cont'd*

3. Shedding of primary teeth
4. Tympanostomy tube insertion
5. Endotracheal intubation
6. Bronchoscopy with a flexible bronchoscope, with or without biopsy
7. Cardiac catheterization
8. Endoscopy with or without gastrointestinal biopsy
9. Cesarean section
10. In the absence of infection for urethral catheterization, dilatation and curettage, uncomplicated vaginal delivery, therapeutic abortion, sterilization procedures, or insertion or removal of intrauterine devices

*This table lists selected conditions but is not meant to be all-inclusive.

†Individuals who have a mitral valve prolapse associated with thickening or redundancy of the valve leaflets may be at increased risk for bacterial endocarditis, particularly men who are 45 years of age or older.

**In addition to prophylactic regimen for genitourinary procedures, antibiotic therapy should be directed against the most likely bacterial pathogen.

‡In patients who have prosthetic heart valves, a previous history of endocarditis, or surgically constructed systemic-pulmonary shunts or conduits, physicians may choose to administer prophylactic antibiotics even for low-risk procedures that involve the lower respiratory, genitourinary, or gastrointestinal tracts.

From Dajani AS et al: *JAMA* 264(22):2919, 1990.

I-45 ANTICOAGULATION IN ATRIAL FIBRILLATION

I. Age < 65	Risk factors*	Warfarin INR 2-3
	No risk factors	ASA or nothing
II. Age 65-75	Risk factors	Warfarin INR 2-3
	No risk factors	Warfarin INR 2-3
III. Age > 75**		Warfarin INR 2-3

*Risk factors are previous TIA or stroke, hypertension, diabetes, clinical coronary artery disease, mitral stenosis, prosthetic heart valve, or thyrotoxicosis.

**Must be weighed against probably age-related bleeding risk.

From Laupacis A et al: *Chest* 108(4):357S, 1995.

CHAPTER II

Endocrinology—Metabolism

II-1 DISORDERS ASSOCIATED WITH HYPOPITUITARISM

I. Primary
- A. Ischemic necrosis of the pituitary
    1. Postpartum (Sheehan's syndrome)
    2. Diabetes mellitus
    3. Other systemic diseases (temporal arteritis, sickle-cell disease and trait, arteriosclerosis, eclampsia)
- B. Pituitary tumors
    1. Primary intrasellar (adenoma, craniopharyngioma)
    2. Parasellar (meningioma, optic nerve glioma)
    3. Metastatic (breast, lung, melanoma)
- C. Aneurysm of intracranial internal carotid artery
- D. Pituitary apoplexy (almost always related to a primary pituitary tumor)
- E. Cavernous sinus thrombosis
- F. Infectious disease (tuberculosis, syphilis, malaria, meningitis, fungal disease)
- G. Infiltrative disease (hemochromatosis)
- H. Immunologic (granulomatous or lymphocytic hypophysitis)
- I. Iatrogenic
    1. Irradiation to nasopharynx
    2. Irradiation to sella
    3. Surgical destruction
- J. Primary empty sella syndrome
- K. Metabolic disorders (chronic renal failure)
- L. Idiopathic (frequently monohormonal)
- M. Genetic (*pit*-1 gene mutation, deletion, GH gene deletions, □-LH mutation, other familial forms)

II. Secondary
- A. Destruction of pituitary stalk
    1. Trauma
    2. Compression by tumor or aneurysm
    3. Iatrogenic (surgical)
- B. Hypothalamic or other central nervous system disease
    1. Inflammatory (sarcoid or other granulomatous disease)
    2. Infiltrative (lipid storage diseases)
    3. Trauma
    4. Toxic (vincristine)
    5. Hormone-induced (glucocorticoids, gonadal steroids)
    6. Tumors (primary, metastatic, lymphomas, leukemia)
    7. Idiopathic (frequently congenital or familial, often restricted to one or two hormones, and may be reversible)
    8. Nutritional (starvation, obesity)
    9. Anorexia nervosa
    10. Psychosocial dwarfism

From Frohman LA. In Felig P, Baxter JD, Frohman LA (eds): *Endocrinology and metabolism,* ed 3, New York, 1995, McGraw-Hill, p. 314.

II-2   CAUSES OF HYPERPROLACTINEMIA

I. Physiologic states
   A. Pregnancy
   B. Nursing (early)
   C. "Stress"
   D. Sleep
   E. Nipple stimulation
   F. Food ingestion
II. Drugs
   A. Dopamine receptor antagonists
      1. Phenothiazines
      2. Butyrophenones
      4. Metoclopramide
      5. Sulpiride
   B. Dopamine-depleting agents (methyldopa, reserpine)
   C. Estrogens
   D. Opiates
III. Disease states
   A. Pituitary tumors
      1. Prolactinomas
      2. Adenomas secreting GH and prolactin
      3. Adenomas secreting ACTH and prolactin (Nelson's syndrome and Cushing's disease)
      4. Nonfunctioning chromophobe adenoma with pituitary stalk compression
   B. Hypothalamic and pituitary stalk disease
      1. Granulomatous diseases (e.g., sarcoidosis)
      2. Craniopharyngiomas and other tumors
      3. Cranial irradiation
      4. Stalk section
      5. Empty sella
      6. Vascular abnormalities including aneurysm
      7. Lymphocytic hypophysitis
      8. Metastatic carcinoma
   C. Primary hypothyroidism
   D. Chronic renal failure
   E. Cirrhosis
   F. Chest wall trauma (including surgery, herpes zoster)
   G. Seizures

From Daniels GH, Martin JB. In Isselbacher KJ et al (eds): *Harrison's principles of internal medicine*, ed 13, New York, 1994, McGraw-Hill, p. 2037.

II-3   CLINICAL FEATURES OF ACROMEGALY

Clinical features	Diagnosis
I. Enlargement of hands, feet, nose, jaw	I. Inappropriately ↑ plasma growth hormone
II. Soft tissue overgrowth	II. Failure of oral glucose to suppress plasma growth hormone
III. Weight gain	
IV. Amenorrhea	III. Abnormal growth hormone response to thyrotropin-releasing hormone
V. Decreased libido	
VI. Arthritis	IV. Hyperglycemia and glucosuria
VII. Hypertrichosis	V. Abnormal skull x-rays (90%)
VIII. Hypertension	VI. Abnormal CT scan
IX. Glucose intolerance	
X. Cardiac dysrhythmias	
XI. Visual field defects	
XII. Paresthesias/peripheral neuropathy	
XIII. Carpal tunnel syndrome	
XIV. Increased sweating	
XV. Voice change	

II-4   FEATURES COMMONLY ASSOCIATED WITH THE PRIMARY EMPTY SELLA SYNDROME

Features	Frequency (%)
Females	83.7
Obesity	78.4
Systemic hypertension	30.5
Benign intracranial hypertension (pseudotumor cerebri)	10.5
CSF rhinorrhea	9.7

From Jordan et al: *Am J Med* 62:569, 1977.

II-5 PHYSIOLOGIC CLASSIFICATION OF GALACTORRHEA

 I. Failure of normal hypothalamic inhibition of prolactin release
    A. Pituitary stalk section
    B. Drugs (phenothiazines, butyrophenones, methyldopa, tricyclic antidepressants, opiates, reserpine, verapamil)
    C. Central nervous system disease, including extrapituitary tumors and null cell adenomas of the pituitary
 II. Enhanced prolactin-releasing factor
    A. Hypothyroidism
    B. Sucking reflex and breast trauma
 III. Autonomous prolactin release
    A. Pituitary tumors
       1. Prolactin-secreting tumors
       2. Mixed growth hormone and prolactin-secreting tumors
       3. Chromophobe adenoma
    B. Ectopic production of human placental lactogen and/or prolactin
       1. Hydatidiform moles and choriocarcinomas
       2. Others (bronchogenic carcinoma and hypernephroma)
 IV. Idiopathic

From Wilson JD. In Isselbacher KJ et al (eds): *Harrison's principles of internal medicine,* ed 13, New York, 1994, McGraw-Hill, p. 2037.

II-6 DIFFERENTIAL DIAGNOSIS OF THE SYNDROME OF INAPPROPRIATE ANTIDIURESIS (SIADH)

 I. Tumors
    A. Bronchogenic carcinoma
    B. Carcinoma of the duodenum
    C. Carcinoma of pancreas
    D. Thymoma
    E. Carcinoma of ureter
    F. Lymphoma
    G. Ewing's sarcoma
    H. Carcinoma of the prostate
    I. Mesothelioma
    J. Carcinoma of the bladder
 II. Nonneoplastic diseases
    A. Trauma
    B. Pulmonary disease

Continued

I-6 DIFFERENTIAL DIAGNOSIS OF THE SYNDROME OF INAPPROPRIATE ANTIDIURESIS (SIADH)—*cont'd*

  1. Pneumonia, bacterial or viral
  2. Cavitation (aspergillosis)
  3. Tuberculosis
  4. Positive-pressure breathing
  5. Lung abscess
  6. Asthma
  7. Pneumothorax
  8. Cystic fibrosis
  C. Central nervous system disorders
  1. Encephalitis or meningitis, bacterial or viral
  2. Head trauma
  3. Brain abscess
  4. Guillain-Barr
  5. Subarachnoid hemorrhage
  6. Acute intermittent porphyria
  7. Peripheral neuropathy
  8. Psychosis
  9. Delirium tremens
  10. Cerebrovascular accident
  11. Cerebral atrophy
  12. Cavernous sinus thrombosis
  13. Hydrocephalus
  14. Rocky Mountain fever
  15. Multiple sclerosis
  D. SIADH in endocrine disease
  1. Myxedema
  E. "Idiopathic" SIADH
III. Drugs
  A. Vasopressin and DDAVP
  B. Oxytocin
  C. Vincristine
  D. Chlorpropamide
  E. Thiazide diuretics
  F. Clofibrate
  G. Carbamazepine
  H. Nicotine
  I. Phenothiazines
  J. Cyclophosphamide
  K. Tricyclic antidepressants
  L. Haloperidol
  M. Monoamine oxidase inhibitors

From Robertson GL. In Felig P, Baxter JD, Frohman LS (eds): *Endocrinology and metabolism*, ed 3, New York, 1995, McGraw-Hill, p.417.

II-7 CAUSES OF HYPERTHYROIDISM

   I. Graves' disease
  II. Thyroiditis
      A. Subacute thyroiditis
      B. Painless thyroiditis
      C. Radiation thyroiditis
 III. Exogenous hyperthyroidism
      A. Iatrogenic
      B. Factitious
      C. Iodine-induced
  IV. Toxic multinodular goiter
   V. Toxic uninodular goiter (thyroid adenoma)
  VI. Ectopic hyperthyroidism (struma ovarii)
 VII. Thyroid carcinoma
VIII. TSH excess
      A. Pituitary thyrotropin
      B. Trophoblastic tumors

From Utiger RD. In Felig P, Baxter JD, Frohman LA (eds): *Endocrinology and metabolism,* ed 3, New York, 1995, McGraw-Hill, p. 467.

II-8 CLINICAL FEATURES OF HYPERTHYROIDISM

Symptoms	Physical signs	Diagnosis
Weight loss	Moist, warm, smooth skin	$\uparrow T_4$
Diarrhea	Tachycardia	$\uparrow$ free T_4
Heat intolerance	Plummer's nails	$\uparrow T_3$
Nervousness	Ocular signs	$\uparrow$ RAI uptake
Excessive sweating	Exophthalmos	$\uparrow T_3$ resin uptake
Emotional	Stare	$\downarrow$ TSH
instability	Lid lag	
Polyphagia	Infrequent blinking	
Fatigue and	Difficulty with convergence	
weakness		
Palpitations	Thyromegaly	
Menstrual	Thyroid bruit	
irregularities	Means-Lerman scratch/high pitched pulmonic sound	
	Atrial dysrhythmias (especially, atrial fibrillation)	
	Heart failure	
	Hepatomegaly	
	Abnormal liver tests	
	Pretibial myxedema	
	Tremor	

II-9   CAUSES OF HYPOTHYROIDISM

 I. Thyroidal hypothyroidism
  A. Insufficient functional tissue
   1. Thyroiditis*
   2. After ^{131}I therapy or thyroidectomy
   3. Thyroid dysgenesis
   4. Infiltrations*
  B. Defective biosynthesis of thyroid hormone
   1. Iodine deficiency*
   2. Congenital defects*
   3. Antithyroid agents*
   4. Iodine excess*
 II. Hypothyrotropic hypothyroidism
  A. Pituitary hypothyroidism
  B. Hypothalamic hypothyroidism
 III. Generalized resistance to thyroid hormones

*Hypothyroidism may be accompanied by goiter in these cases.

From Utiger RD. In Felig P, Baxter JD, Frohman LA (eds): *Endocrinology and metabolism,* ed 3, New York, 1995, McGraw-Hill, p. 493.

II-10   CLINICAL FEATURES OF HYPOTHYROIDISM

Symptoms	Signs	Diagnosis
Lethargy	Deep hoarse voice	↓ T_4
Constipation	Periorbital puffiness	↓ Free T_4
Cold intolerance	Pretibial myxedema	↓ T_3 resin uptake
Menorrhagia	Macroglossia	↑ TSH
Mental slowing	Decreased auditory acuity	↑ Cholesterol
Motor slowing	Pericardial effusion	↑ LDH
Anorexia	Cardiomegaly	↑ CPK
Weight gain	Ileus	↑ SGOT
Dry skin	Psychosis	
Dry brittle hair	Cerebellar ataxia	
Muscle aches	Prolonged relaxation phase of deep tendon reflexes	
	Stupor or coma	
	Bradycardia	
	Ascites	
	Loss of outer third of eyebrows	
	Carpal tunnel syndrome	

II-11   METABOLIC CAUSES OF PSYCHIATRIC DISTURBANCES IN OLDER PERSONS

I. Delirium
   A. Hypoxemia
   B. Electrolyte disturbances
   C. Acid-base abnormalities
   D. Uremia
   E. Hepatic failure
   F. Thyroid disorders
   G. Hypoglycemia
   H. Hypoparathyroidism
   I. Hyperparathyroidism
   J. Hypoadrenalism
   K. Hypopituitarism
   L. Isolated ACTH deficiency
   M. Exogenous corticosteroids
   N. Thiamine deficiency
   O. Pellagra
   P. Porphyria

II. Depression
   A. Hypokalemia
   B. Apathetic thyrotoxicosis
   C. Hypothyroidism
   D. Diabetes mellitus
   E. Hyperparathyroidism
   F. Cushing's disease
   G. Addisson's disease
   H. Malnutrition
   I. Pernicious anemia
   J. Folate deficiency
   K. Impotence

III. Dementia
   A. Hypoxemia
   B. Electrolyte disturbances
   C. Hyperlipidemia
   D. Hypothyroidism
   E. Hypoglycemia
   F. Diabetes mellitus
   G. Hypoparathyroidism
   H. Hyperparathyroidism
   I. Hypoadrenalism
   J. Malnutrition
   K. Pernicious anemia
   L. Folate deficiency
   M. Dehydration

From Morely JE. In Felig P, Baxter JD, Frohman LA (eds): *Endocrinology and metabolism,* ed 3, New York, 1995, McGraw-Hill, p. 1815.

II-12   CAUSES OF INFERTILITY AND THEIR APPROXIMATE INCIDENCE (%)

I. Male factors
   A. Decreased spermatozoa production
      1. Varicocele
      2. Testicular failure
      3. Endocrine disorders
      4. Cryptorchidism
      5. Stress, smoking, caffeine, nicotine, recreational drugs
   B. Ductal obstruction
      1. Epididymal (postinfection)
      2. Congenital absence of vas deferens
      3. Ejaculatory duct (postinfection)
      4. Postvasectomy
   C. Inability to deliver sperm into vagina
      2. Hypospadias
      3. Sexual problems (i.e., impotence), medical or psychological
   D. Abnormal semen
      1. Infection
      2. Abnormal volume
      3. Abnormal viscosity
   E. Immunologic factors
      1. Sperm-immobilizing antibodies
      2. Sperm-agglutinating antibodies
II. Female factors
   A. Fallopian tube pathology (20 to 30%)
      1. Pelvic inflammatory disease or puerperal infection
      2. Congenital anomalies
      3. Endometriosis
      4. Secondary to past peritonitis of nongenital origin
   B. Amenorrhea and anovulation (15%)
   C. Minor ovulatory disturbances (<5%)
   D. Cervical and uterine factors (10%)
   E. Vaginal factors (<5%)
      1. Congenital absence of vagina
      2. Imperforate hymen
      3. Vaginismus
      4. Vaginitis
   F. Immunologic factors (<5%)
      1. Sperm-immobilizing antibodies
      2. Sperm-agglutinating antibodies
   G. Nutritional and metabolic factors (5%)
      1. Thyroid disorders
      2. Diabetes mellitus
      3. Severe nutritional disturbances
III. Idiopathic or unexplained (<10%)

From Rebar RW. In Bennett JC, Plum F (eds): *Cecil textbook of medicine*, ed 20, Philadelphia, 1996, WB Saunders, p. 1308.

II-13   STATES ASSOCIATED WITH DECREASED PERIPHERAL CONVERSION OF T4 TO T3

I. Physiologic
   A. Fetal and early neonatal life
   B. Old age
II. Pathologic
   A. Fasting
   B. Malnutrition
   C. Systemic illness
   D. Physical trauma
   E. Postoperative state
   F. Drugs (propylthiouracil, dexamethasone, propranolol, amiodarone)
   G. Radiographic contrast agents (ipodate, ipanoate)

From Wortofsky L. In Isselbacher KJ et al (eds): *Harrison's principles of internal medicine,* ed 13, New York, 1994, McGraw-Hill, p. 1933.

II-14   ADRENAL CORTICAL INSUFFICIENCY

I. Etiology of primary adrenocortical insufficiency
   A. Idiopathic/autoimmune ($\cong$80%)
   B. Tuberculosis ($\cong$20%)
   C. Miscellaneous ($\cong$1%)
      1. (A) Hemorrhage: sepsis, anticoagulants, coagulopathy, trauma, surgery, pregnancy, neonatal
         (B) Infarction: thrombosis, embolism arteritis
      2. Fungal infection: histoplasmosis, coccidioidomycosis, blastomycosis, torulosis, cryptococcosis, paracoccidiomycosis
      3. Metastatic neoplasm
      4. Lymphoma
      5. Amyloidosis
      6. Sarcoidosis
      7. Hemochromatosis
      8. Surgery: bilateral adrenalectomy
      9. Enzyme inhibitors: metyrapone, aminoglutethimide, trilostane, ketoconazole, etomidate
      10. Cytotoxic agents: mitotane
      11. Congenital: adrenal hyperplasia, hypoplasia, familial glucocorticoid deficiency, adrenal leukodystrophy
      12. Acquired immunodeficiency syndrome (AIDS)
      13. Irradiation

Continued

II-14   ADRENAL CORTICAL INSUFFICIENCY—*cont'd*

II. Clinical disorders associated with idiopathic adrenocortical insufficiency (%)
   A. Primary ovarian failure: 23%
   B. Thyroid
      1. Thyrotoxicosis: 7%
      2. Hypothyroidism/chronic thyroiditis: 9%
   C. Diabetes mellitus: 12%
   D. Vitiligo: 9%
   E. Hypoparathyroidism: 6%
   F. Pernicious anemia: 4%

From Irvine WJ, Barnes EW: Adrenocortical insufficiency, *Clin Endocrinol Metab* 1:549-594, 1972; Miller WL, Tyrrell JB. In Felig P, Baxter JD, Frohman LA (eds): *Endocrinology and metabolism*, ed 3, New York, 1995, McGraw-Hill, p. 642.

II-15   CLINICAL FEATURES OF ADDISON'S DISEASE

Symptoms and physical signs	Diagnosis
I. Anorexia	I. ↓ plasma cortisol
II. Weakness and easy fatigability	A. Little increase after synthetic ACTH
III. Nausea and vomiting	B. ↑ ACTH levels with primary adrenal failure
IV. Weight loss	
V. Salt craving	II. ↓ urinary 17-hydroxy and 17-ketosteroid
VI. Diarrhea	III. Hyponatremia
VII. Postural hypotension	IV. Hyperkalemia
VIII. Hyperpigmentation	V. Anemia
IX. Personality changes	VI. Eosinophilia
X. Decrease in axillary and pubic hair	VII. Reduction in heart size
XI. Muscle and joint pains	VII. Hypercalcemia (rare; with adrenal crisis)
XII. Amenorrhea	

II-16 CUSHING'S SYNDROME

I. Classification and etiology
- A. ACTH dependent
    1. Cushing's disease: 68%
    2. Ectopic ACTH syndrome: 15%
- B. ACTH independent
    1. Adrenal adenoma: 9%
    2. Adrenal carcinoma: 8%

TOTAL: 100%

From Huff TA. Clinical syndromes related to disorders of adrenocorticotrophic hormone. In Allen MB, Makesh VB (eds): *The pituitary: A current review,* New York, 1977, Academic Press, pp. 153-168.

II. Tumors most frequently causing the ectopic ACTH syndrome
- A. Oat cell carcinoma of the lung
- B. Pancreatic islet cell carcinoma
- C. Carcinoid tumors (lung, gut, thymus, pancreas, ovary)
- D. Thyroid medullary carcinoma
- E. Pheochromocytoma and related tumors

From Miller WL, Tyrrell JB. In Felig P, Baxter JD, Frohman LA (eds): *Endocrinology and metabolism,* ed 3, New York, 1995, McGraw-Hill, p. 663.

11-17 CLINICAL FEATURES OF CUSHING'S SYNDROME

Clinical features	Diagnosis
I. Typical facial feature and habitus	I. Plasma cortisol usually ↑
II. Weight gain	A. No suppression with pm dexamethasone
III. Weakness and easy fatigability	II. ↑ urinary 17-hydroxycorticoid; free cortisol ↑
IV. Amenorrhea	III. Suppression of plasma cortisol and urinary hydrycorticoids by low or high dose dexamethasone
V. Personality changes	IV. Mild leukocytosis
VI. Polyuria, polydipsia	V. Eosinopenia
	VI. Hypokalemic alkalosis
	VII. Hyperglycemia
	VIII. CT scan may be of value
VII. Hypertension	
VIII. Hirsutism, striae, ecchymosis	
IX. Edema	
X. Clitoral hypertrophy	

II-18   SYNDROME OF PRIMARY ALDOSTERONISM

I. Etiology
- A. Aldosterone-producing adenoma
- B. Adrenocortical hyperplasia
  1. Idiopathic aldosteronism (aldosterone production-nonsuppressible)
  2. Indeterminate aldosteronism (aldosterone production-suppressible)
  3. Glucocorticoid-suppressible aldosteronism
  4. Surgically remediable aldosteronism (?)
- C. Adrenocortical carcinoma

II. Clinical features
- A. Symptoms and signs
  1. Hypertension
  2. Muscle weakness
  3. Polyuria
  4. Polydipsia
- B. Diagnosis
  1. Hypokalemia
  2. Hypernatremia (occasional)
  3. Alkaline to neutral urine pH
  4. Metabolic alkalosis
  5. Hyperglycemia
  6. Failure of plasma renin to rise normally
     a. diuretics
     b. upright
     c. sodium depletion
  7. Failure to suppress serum aldosterone with saline infusion
  8. CT scan may be helpful

II-19 CLASSIFICATION OF SECONDARY HYPERALDOSTERONISM

Primary abnormality	Potassium loss	Edema	Hyper-tension	Effect of sodium load
Extrarenal sodium loss Hemorrhage Thermal stress Gastrointestinal loss	Absent	Absent	Absent	Repairs deficit
Sodium restriction	Absent	Absent	Absent	Repairs deficit
Abnormal distribution of sodium excess Congestive heart failure Nephrotic syndrome Cirrhosis with ascites Idiopathic edema	Present	Present	Absent	Worsens edema
Abnormal renal Electrolyte loss Slat-losing renal disease Bartter's syndrome Diuretic abuse Renal tubular acidosis	Present	Absent	Absent	Variable
Other renal lesions Renal artery stenosi Unilateral renal ischemia Accelerated hypertension	Present	Absent	Present	May worsen hyper-tension
Other renal lesions Renin-secreting tumor Chronic renal failure*	Present	Absent	Present	May worsen
Excessive potassium intake	Present	Absent	Absent	May facilitate haluresis
Luteal phase of menstrual cycle and pregnancy	Absent	May be present	Usually present	Suppresses renin and aldosterone

*Exception; no potassium loss.

From Stocking JR. Mineralocorticoid excess. In James VHT (ed): *The adrenal gland,* New York, 1979, Raven Press, pp. 197-242.

From Miller WL, Tyrrell JB. In Felig P, Baxter JD, Frohman LA (eds): *Endocrinology and metabolism,* ed 3, New York, 1995, McGraw-Hill, p. 679.

II-20 CAUSES OF HYPOMAGNESEMIA AND MAGNESIUM DEPLETION

I. Decreased intake and/or absorption
   A. Protein-calorie malnutrition
   B. Losses of gastrointestinal fluids
   C. Malabsorption syndromes
   D. Primary hypomagnesemia
   E. Parenteral hyperalimentation without adequate magnesium
II. Renal losses
   A. Osmotic diuresis; mannitol, glucose, urea
   B. After relief of obstruction or resolution of acute tubular necrosis
   C. After renal transplant
   D. Drugs
      1. Diuretics
      2. Cisplatin
      3. Aminoglycosides
      4. Amphotericin
      5. Digoxin
      6. Pentamidine
      7. Theophylline toxicity
      8. Cyclosporine
   E. ECF expansion, Bartter's syndrome, hyperaldosteronism
   F. Congenital, hereditary wasting
III. Miscellaneous disorders
   A. Chronic alcoholism
   B. Diabetic ketoacidosis/diabetes mellitus
   C. Primary hyperparathyroidism
   D. After parathyroidectomy
   E. Chronic hypoparathyroidism
   F. Hyperthyroidism
   G. SIADH
   H. Hypoalbuminemia
   I. Dialysis
   J. Excessive lactation
   K. Pancreatitis

From Strewler GJ, Rosenblatt M. In Felig P, Baxter JD, Frohman LA (eds): *Endocrinology and metabolism,* ed 3, New York, 1995, McGraw-Hill, p. 1496.

II-21 CLASSIFICATION OF DIABETES MELLITUS

I. Spontaneous diabetes mellitus
   A. Type I or insulin-dependent diabetes (formerly called juvenile-onset diabetes)
   B. Type II or insulin-independent diabetes (formerly called maturity-onset diabetes)
II. Secondary diabetes
   A. Pancreatic disease (pancreoprival diabetes, e.g., pancreatectomy, pancreatic insufficiency, hemochromatosis)
   B. Hormonal: excess secretion of counterregulatory hormones (e.g., acromegaly, Cushing's syndrome, pheochromocytoma)
   C. Drug induced (e.g., potassium-losing diuretics, contrainsulin hormones, psychoactive agents, phenytoin)
   D. Associated with complex genetic syndrome (e.g., ataxia telangiectasia, Lawrence-Moon-Biedl syndrome, myotonic dystrophy, Friedreich's ataxia)
III. Impaired glucose tolerance (formerly called chemical diabetes, asymptomatic diabetes, latent diabetes, and subclinical diabetes): normal fasting plasma glucose, and 2-hour value on glucose tolerance test >140 mg/dl but <200 mg/dl
IV. Gestational diabetes: glucose intolerance that has its onset in pregnancy

From National Diabetes Data Group: Diabetes 28:1039, 1979. Adapted from Felig P, Bergman M. In Felig P, Baxter JD, Frohman LA (eds): *Endocrinology and metabolism*, ed 3, New York, 1995, McGraw-Hill, p. 1157.

II-22 PRECIPITATING FACTORS IN DIABETIC KETOACIDOSIS

I. Infection
   A. Urinary tract
   B. Pneumonias
   C. Cellulitis
   D. Periodontal
   E. Central nervous system
   F. Septicemia
II. Metabolic/endocrine
   A. Uremia
   B. Hypothyroidism
   C. Cushing's syndrome
III. Dietary indiscretion
IV. Not taking insulin
V. Pregnancy
VI. Myocardial infarction
VII. CVA
VIII. Drugs
   A. Thiazides
   B. Corticosteroids
IX. Acute pancreatitis
X. Excessive alcohol consumption

II-23 MAJOR CAUSES OF FASTING HYPOGLYCEMIA

I. Conditions primarily due to underproduction of glucose
   A. Hormone deficiencies
      1. Hypopituitarism
      2. Adrenal insufficiency
      3. Catecholamine deficiency
      4. Glucagon deficiency
   B. Enzyme defects
      1. Glucose 6-phosphatase
      2. Liver phosphorylase
      3. Pyruvate carboxylase
      4. Phosphoenolpyruvate carboxykinase
      5. Fructose 1,6-diphosphatase
      6. Glycogen synthetase
   C. Substrate deficiency
      1. Ketotic hypoglycemia of infancy
      2. Severe malnutrition, muscle wasting
      3. Late pregnancy
   D. Acquired liver disease
      1. Hepatic congestion
      2. Severe hepatitis
      3. Cirrhosis
      4. Uremia
      5. Hypothermia
   E. Drugs
      1. Alcohol
      2. Propranolol
      3. Salicylates
II. Conditions primarily due to overutilization of glucose
   A. Hyperinsulinism
      1. Insulinoma
      2. Exogenous insulin
      3. Sulfonylureas
      4. Immune disease with insulin or insulin receptor antibodies
      5. Drugs: quinine, disopyramide, pentamidine
      6. Endotoxic shock
   B. Appropriate insulin levels
      1. Extrapancreatic tumors
      2. Carnitine deficiency
      3. Cachexia with fat depletion
      4. Deficiency in enzymes of fat oxidation
      5. 3-Hydroxy-3-methylglutaryl-CoA lyase deficiency

From Foster DW, Rubenstein AH. In Isselbacher KJ et al (eds): *Harrison's principles of internal medicine,* ed 13, New York, 1994, McGraw-Hill, p. 2002.

II-24   INSULIN RESISTANT STATES

I. Prereceptor resistance
   A. Mutated insulins
   B. Anti-insulin antibodies
II. Receptor and postreceptor resistance
   A. Obesity
   B. Type A syndrome (absent or dysfunctional receptor)
   C. Type B syndrome (antibody to insulin receptor)
   D. Lipodystrophic states (partial or generalized)
   E. Leprechaunism
   F. Ataxia–telangiectasia
   G. Rabson-Mendenhall syndrome
   H. Werner syndrome
   I. Alström's syndrome
   J. Pineal hyperplasia syndrome

From Foster DW. In Isselbacher KJ et al (eds): *Harrison's principles of internal medicine,* ed 13, New York, 1994, McGraw-Hill, p. 1998.

II-25 A CLASSIFICATION OF THE OBESITIES

I. Etiologic
  A. Hypothalamic dysfunction
    1. Tumors
    2. Inflammation
    3. Trauma and surgical injury
    4. Increased intracranial pressure
    5. Functional changes causing hyperinsulinemia?
  B. Endocrine
    1. Glucocorticoid excess (Cushing's syndrome)
    2. Thyroid hormone deficiency (hypothyroidism)
    3. Hypopituitarism
    4. Gonadal deficiency (primary and secondary hypogo-
       nadism)
    5. Hyperinsulinism (insulinoma, excess exogenous insulin)
  C. Genetic
    1. Inherited predisposition to obesity
    2. Genetic syndromes associated with obesity:
      a. Prader-Willi syndrome
      b. Alström's syndrome
      c. Laurence-Moon-Bardet-Biedl syndrome
      d. Stewart-Morel-Morgagni syndrome (hyperostosis fron-
         talis internal)
      e. Down's syndrome
      f. Pseudo- and pseudo-pseudo-hypoparathyroidism
  D. Nutritional
    1. Maternal nutritional factors?
    2. Infant feeding practices?
    3. Excess colonic intake during adulthood
  E. Drugs
    1. Phenothiazines
    2. Insulin
    3. Corticosteroids
    4. Cyproheptadine
    5. Tricyclic antidepressants
II. Anatomic
  A. Hypercellular-hypertrophic: early age of onset, severe obesity
  B. Hypertrophic-normal cellular; adult onset, milder obesity
III. Contributory factors
  A. Familial influences
  B. Physical inactivity
  C. Dietary factors: eating patterns, type of diet
  D. Socioeconomic
  E. Educational
  F. Cultural-ethnic
  G. Psychologic

From Salans LB. In Felig P, Baxter JD, Broadus AE et al (eds): *Endocrinology and metabolism,* ed 2, New York, 1987, McGraw-Hill, p. 1225.

II-26   CAUSES OF HYPERCALCEMIA

I. Primary hyperparathyroidism
   A. Sporadic
   B. Clinical variants and familial syndromes
   C. After renal transplantation
II. Neoplastic diseases
   A. Local osteolysis (breast, lung, kidney, etc)
   B. Humoral hypercalcemia of malignancy
   C. Hematologic malignancy (multiple myeloma, lymphoma, leukemia, etc.)
III. Endocrinopathies
   A. Thyrotoxicosis
   B. Adrenal insufficiency
   C. Pheochromocytoma
   D. VIP-oma syndrome
   E. Acromegaly
IV. Medications
   A. Thiazide diuretics
   B. Vitamins A and D
   C. Milk alkali syndrome
   D. Lithium
   E. Estrogens, androgens, tamoxifen
V. Sarcoidosis and other granulomatous diseases
VI. Miscellaneous conditions
   A. Immobilization
   B. Acute renal failure
   C. Idiopathic hypercalcemia of infancy
   D. Serum protein abnormalities
   E. Familial hypocalciuric hypercalcemia
   F. Dehydration
   G. ICU hypercalcemia

From Strewler GJ, Rosenblatt M. In Felig P, Baxter JD, Frohman LA (eds): *Endocrinology and metabolism,* ed 3, New York, 1995, McGraw-Hill, p. 1450.

II-27   MEDICAL COMPLICATIONS OF OBESITY

I. Cardiovascular
   A. Coronary artery disease
   B. Myocardial infarction
   C. Congestive heart failure
   D. Sudden death
   E. Cerebrovascular accidents
   F. Hypertension
   G. Left ventricular hypertrophy
II. Metabolic
   A. Hyperlipidemia
   B. Insulin resistance
   C. Non-insulin-dependent diabetes mellitus
   D. Cholesterol gallstones
III. Cancer
   A. Males: colon, rectum prostate
   B. Females: breast, ovary, endometrium, cervix, gallbladder, bile ducts
IV. Hormonal
   A. Menstrual abnormalities
   B. Hyperandrogenism
   C. Hirsutism
   D. Acanthosis nigricans
   E. Polycystic ovaries
   F. Decreased six hormone-binding globulin
   G. Increased estrogens
   H. Decreased testosterone in males
   I. Decreased growth hormone
   J. Decreased prolactin responsiveness
   K. Enhanced cortisol production
V. Rheumatic (osteoarthritis)
VI. Pulmonary
   A. Decreased functional reserve capacity
   B. Decreased total lung capacity
   C. Decreased expiratory reserve volume
   D. Decreased maximum expiratory flow rate in males
   E. Increased residual volume
   F. Increased diffusing capacity
   G. Sleep apnea and obesity hypoventilation syndrome

From Amatruda JM, Welle S. In Felig P, Baxter JD, Frohman LA, (eds): *Endocrinology and metabolism,* ed 3, New York, 1995, McGraw-Hill, p. 1274.

II-28 CAUSES OF HYPOCALCEMIA

I. Hypoparathyroidism
   A. Surgical
   B. Idiopathic
   C. Neonatal
   D. Familial
   E. Deposition of metals (iron, copper, aluminum)
   F. Postradiation
   G. Infiltrative
   H. Functional (in hypomagnesemia)
II. Resistance to PTH action
   A. Pseudohypoparathyroidism
   B. Renal insufficiency
   C. Medications that block osteoblastic bone resorption
      1. Plicamycin (mithramycin)
      2. Calcitonin
      3. Bisphosphonates
III. Failure to produce 1 alpha, 25(OH)$_2$D normally
   A. Vitamin D deficiency
   B. Hereditary 1 alpha-hydroxylase deficiency
   C. Renal insufficiency
IV. Resistance to 1 alpha, 25(OH)$_2$ action: hereditary 1 alpha, 25(OH)$_2$D-resistant rickets
V. Acute complexation of deposition of calcium
   A. Hyperphosphatemia
      1. Crush injury
      2. Rapid tumor lysis
      3. Parenteral phosphate administration
      4. Excessive enteral phosphate (oral, phosphate-containing enemas)
      5. Acute pancreatitis
      6. Citrated blood transfusion
      7. Rapid excessive skeletal mineralization
         a. Hungry bones syndrome
         b. Osteoblastic metastases
         c. Vitamin D therapy for vitamin D deficiency
VI. Miscellaneous
   A. Intestinal malabsorption
   B. Hepatic and biliary disorders
   C. Anticonvulsant therapy
   D. Hypoalbuminemia

From Strewler GJ, Rosenblatt M. In Felig P, Baxter JD, Frohman LA, (eds): *Endocrinology and metabolism,* ed 3, New York, 1995, McGraw-Hill, p. 1478.

II-29 CLASSIFICATION OF OSTEOMALACIA AND RICKETS

I. Reduction of circulating vitamin D metabolites
   A. Inadequate ultraviolet light exposure and inadequate dietary vitamin D
   B. Vitamin D malabsorption
      1. Small intestinal disease
      2. Pancreatic insufficiency
      3. Insufficient bile salts
   C. Abnormal vitamin D metabolism
      1. Liver disease
      2. Chronic renal failure
      3. Drugs (anticonvulsants, glutethimide)
      4. Mesenchymal tumors, prostatic cancer
      5. Vitamin D-dependent rickets (25-hydroxyvitamin D-1A-hydroxylase deficiency)
   D. Renal loss (nephrotic syndrome)
II. Peripheral resistance to vitamin D
   A. Vitamin D-dependent rickets, type II
   B. Anticonvulsant drugs
   C. Chronic renal failure
III. Hypophosphatemia
   A. Renal phosphate wasting
      1. Hypophosphatemic wasting
         a. Familial X-linked
         b. Autosomal recessive
         c. Sporadic
      2. Hypophosphatemic osteomalacia
         a. Familial X-linked
         b. Sporadic
      3. Fanconi's syndrome
      4. Mesenchymal tumors, fibrous dysplasias, epidermal nevus syndrome, prostatic cancer
      5. Primary hyperparathyroidism
      6. Familial renal phosphate leak with hypercalciuria, nephrolithiasis, osteomalacia, and rickets
   B. Malnutrition
   C. Malabsorption due to gastrointestinal disease or phosphate-binding antacids
   D. Chronic dialysis
IV. Miscellaneous
   A. Inhibitors of calcification
      1. Sodium fluoride
      2. Disodium etidronate
   B. Calcium deficiency
   C. Hypophosphatasia
   D. Fibrogenesis imperfecta ossium
   E. Hypoparathyroidism
   F. Systemic acidosis
   G. Total parenteral nutrition

From Singer FR. In Felig P, Baxter JD, Frohman LA (eds): *Endocrinology and metabolism,* ed 3, New York, 1995, McGraw-Hill, p. 1525.

II-30   CLASSIFICATION OF OSTEOPOROSIS

I. Aging
II. Endocrine abnormality
   A. Estrogen deficiency
   B. Testosterone deficiency
   C. Steroid excess
      1. Cushing's syndrome
      2. Corticosteroid excess
   D. Thyrotoxicosis
   E. Primary hyperparathyroidism
   F. Diabetes mellitus
III. Nutritional abnormality
   A. Vitamin C deficiency
   B. Protein deficiency
   C. Calcium deficiency
   D. Malabsorption
IV. Immobilization or weightlessness
V. Hematologic malignancy
   A. Multiple myeloma
   B. Leukemia
   C. Lymphoma
VI. Genetic
   A. Osteogenesis imperfecta
   B. Ehlers-Danlos syndrome
   C. Homocystinuria
   D. Marfan syndrome
   E. Menkes' syndrome
   F. Lysinuric protein intolerance
VII. Miscellaneous disorders
   A. Systemic mastocytosis
   B. Heparin therapy
   C. Rheumatoid arthritis
   D. Chronic liver disease (especially primary biliary cirrhosis)
   E. Juvenile osteoporosis
   F. Idiopathic
   G. Chronic hypophosphatemia
   H. Chronic alcoholism
   I. Cigarettes
   J. Renal hypercalciuria
   K. Anticonvulsant therapy
   L. Chronic obstructive pulmonary disease

From Singer FR, Frohman LA. In Felig P, Baxter JD, Frohman LA (eds): *Endocrinology and metabolism,* ed 3, New York, 1995, McGraw-Hill, p. 1534.

II-31 CAUSES OF HIRSUTISM IN FEMALES

I. Familial
II. Idiopathic
III. Ovarian
    A. Polycystic ovaries; hilus-cell hyperplasia
    B. Tumor; arrhenoblastoma, hilus cell, adrenal rest
IV. Adrenal
    A. Congenital adrenal hyperplasia
    B. Noncongenital adrenal hyperplasia (Cushing's)
    C. Tumor; virilizing carcinoma or adenoma
V. Drugs: minoxidil, androgens

From Williams GH, Dluhy RG. In Isselbacher KJ et al (eds): *Harrison's principles of internal medicine,* ed 13, New York, 1994, McGraw-Hill, p. 1969.

II-32 CAUSES OF AMENORRHEA

I. Primary amenorrhea
    A. Gonadal dysgenesis (Turner's syndrome)
    B. Pure gonadal dysgenesis (XX gonadal dysgenesis)
    C. Swyer's syndrome (XY gonadal dysgenesis)
    D. Testicular feminization
    E. Pelvic anatomic abnormalities
        1. Uterine agenesis
        2. Cervical stenosis
        3. Intrauterine synechiae
        4. Imperforate hymen
    F. Hypothalamic and pituitary tumors
        1. Craniopharyngioma
        2. Dysgerminoma
        3. Prolactin-secreting tumors
    G. Systemic illness
    H. Weight loss
    I. Stress
    J. Athletic training
    K. "Physiologic delay" of puberty
    L. Hypogonadotropic hypogonadism (Kallmann's syndrome)
II. Secondary amenorrhea
    A. Premature menopause
    B. Autoimmune ovarial failure
    C. "Resistant" ovary syndrome
    D. Stress, weight loss, exercise
    E. Systemic disease
    F. Prolactin-secreting pituitary microadenoma
    G. Destructive or infiltrative hypothalamic or pituitary lesions
    H. Virilizing syndromes
        1. Idiopathic hirsutism
        2. Polycystic ovarian disease
        3. Attenuated forms of congenital adrenal hyperplasia
        4. Insulin resistance
        5. Loss of endometrium (Asherman's syndrome)

From *Endocrinology and metabolism,* MKSAP VII, American College of Physicians, pp. 220-221, 1986.

II-33   DIFFERENTIAL DIAGNOSIS OF GYNECOMASTIA

I. Physiologic gynecomastia
   A. Newborn
   B. Adolescence
   C. Aging
II. Pathologic gynecomastia
   A. Deficient production or action of testosterone
      1. Congenital anorchia
      2. Klinefelter's syndrome
      3. Androgen resistance (testicular feminization and Reifenstein's syndrome)
      4. Defects in testosterone synthesis
      5. Secondary testicular failure (viral orchitis, trauma castration, neurologic and granulomatous diseases, renal failure)
   B. Increased estrogen production
      1. Estrogen secretion
         a. True hermaphroditism
         b. Testicular tumors
         c. Carcinoma of the lung and other tumors producing HCG
      2. Increased substrate for peripheral aromatase
         a. Adrenal disease
         b. Liver disease
         c. Malnutrition
         d. Hyperthyroidism
      3. Increase in extraglandular aromatase
   C. Drugs
      1. Inhibitors of testosterone synthesis and/or action (spironolactone, cimetidine, alkylating agents, cisplatin, metronidazole, ketoconazole, flutamide, etomidate).
      2. Estrogens (diethylstilbestrol, birth control pills, digitalis, cosmetics or foods containing estrogen, phytoestrogens)
      3. Drugs that enhance endogenous estrogen secretion (clomiphene, gonadotropins)
      4. Unknown mechanisms (busulfan, isoniazid, methyldopa, tricyclic antidepressants, D-penicillamine, diazepam, marijuana, heroin, omeprazole, calcium channel blockers, angiotensin-converting enzyme inhibitors)
   D. Idiopathic

From Wilson JD. In Isselbacher KJ et al (eds): *Harrison's principles of internal medicine,* ed 13, New York, 1994, McGraw-Hill, p. 2038.

II-34   CLASSIFICATION OF HYPERLIPIDEMIAS BASED ON LIPOPROTEIN CONCENTRATIONS*

Type	Lipoprotein abnormality	Lipid profiles	Typical values mg/dl
I	Chylomicrons markedly ↑VLDL and LDL both normal or low	Chol ↑ Tg · ↑↑	320 4000
IIa	LDL ↑, VLDL normal	Chol ↑ Tg N	370 90
IIb	LDL ↑, VLDL ↑	Chol ↑ Tg ↑	350 400
III	Abnormal cholesterol-enriched VLDL present in excess	Chol ↑ Tg ↑	500 700
IV	VLDL ↑, LDL normal	Chol N Tg ↑	220
V	Chylomicrons markedly ↑, VLDL ↑, LDL normal or low	Chol ↑ Tg ↑↑	700 5000

II-35   PRIMARY VS. SECONDARY HYPERLIPIDEMIAS

I. Primary: genetic
II. Secondary:
  A. Diet: excessive cholesterol, saturated fat, or calories
  B. Diabetes mellitus
  C. Alcohol
  D. Hypothyroidism
  E. Nephrotic syndrome
  F. Chronic renal failure
  G. Biliary obstruction; primary biliary cirrhosis
  H. Dysglobulinemia; multiple myeloma
  I. Glycogen storage disease
  J. Acute intermittent porphyria
  K. Cushing's syndrome
  L. Anorexia nervosa
  M. Hepatoma
  N. Drug-induced: corticosteroids, estrogens, thiazides, beta blockers, 13-*cis*-retinoic acid (isotretinoin, Accutane)
  O. Autoimmune disease

From Illingworth DR, Duell PB, Connor WE. In Felig P, Baxter JD, Frohman LA (eds): *Endocrinology and metabolism*, ed 3, New York, 1995, McGraw-Hill, p. 1330.

II-36   SOME ORGANIC CAUSES OF ERECTILE IMPOTENCE IN MEN

I. Neurologic diseases
   A. Anterior temporal lobe lesions
   B. Diseases of the spinal cord
   C. Loss of sensory input (tabes dorsalis, disease of the dorsal root ganglia)
   D. Disease of nervi erigentes
      1. Radical prostatectomy and cystectomy
      2. Rectosigmoid operations
   E. Diabetic autonomic neuropathy, various polyneuropathies

II. Endocrine causes
   A. Testicular failure (primary or secondary)
   B. Hyperprolactinemia
   C. Thyroid disease
   D. Cushing's disease

III. Penile diseases
   A. Peyronie's disease
   B. Previous priapism
   C. Penile trauma

IV. Vascular disease
   A. Aortic occlusions (Leriche syndrome)
   B. Atherosclerotic occlusion or stenosis of the pudendal and/or cavernosa arteris
   C. Arterial damage from pelvic radiation
   D. Venous leak
   E. Disease of the sinusoidal spaces

V. Drugs
   A. Antiandrogens
      1. Histamine blockers (e.g., cimetidine, hydroxyzine)
      2. Spironolactone
      3. Ketoconazole
      4. Finasteride
   B. Antihypertensives
      1. Centrally acting sympatholytics (e.g., clonidine and methyldopa)
      2. Peripheral acting sympatholytics (e.g., guanadrel)
      3. Beta blockers
      4. Thiazides
   C. Anticholinergics
   D. Antidepressants
      1. Tricyclic antidepressants
      2. Monoamine oxidase inhibitors
   E. Antipsychotics
      1. Chlorpromazine
      2. Haloperidol
      3. Thioridazine
      4. Metoclopramide

Continued

II-36   SOME ORGANIC CAUSES OF ERECTILE IMPOTENCE IN MEN—*cont'd*

   F. Central nervous system depressants
      1. Sedatives (e.g., barbiturates)
      2. Antianxiety drugs (e.g., diazepam)
   G. Drugs of habituation or addiction
      1. Alcohol
      2. Methadone
      3. Heroin
      4. Tobacco
   H. Other
      1. Cytotoxic agents
      2. NSAIDs
      3. Estrogens
      4. Digoxin
      5. Anticonvulsants

From Wilson JD, McConnell JD, et al. In Isselbacher KJ et al (eds): *Harrison's principles of internal medicine*, ed 13, New York, 1994, McGraw-Hill, p. 263.

II-37   HYPOPHOSPHATEMIA

   I. Increased excretion of phosphorus in the urine
     A. Primary hyperparathyroidism
     B. Secondary hyperparathyroidism
     C. Renal tubular defects
     D. Diuretic phase of acute tubular necrosis
     E. Postobstructive diuresis
     F. Postrenal transplantation
     G. ECF volume expansion
   II. Abnormalities of vitamin D metabolism
     A. Vitamin D-deficient rickets
     B. Familial hypophosphatemic rickets
     C. Vitamin D-dependent rickets
     D. Hypophosphatemia associated with tumors
   III. Decrease in gastrointestinal absorption of phosphorus
     A. Malabsorption
     B. Malnutrition-starvation
     C. Administration of phosphate binders
   IV. Miscellaneous causes
     A. Diabetes mellitus: during treatment for ketoacidosis
     B. Severe respiratory alkalosis
     C. Recovery phase of malnutrition
     D. Alcohol withdrawal
     E. Toxic shock syndrome
     F. Leukemia, lymphoma
     G. Severe burns

From Slatopolsky E, Klahr S. In Schrier R, Gottschalk MD (eds): *Diseases of the kidney*, ed 5, Boston, 1993, Little Brown, p. 2604.

II-38   COMPLICATIONS OF CORTICOSTEROID THERAPY

I. Stigmata of hypercorticism
  A. Acne
  B. Hirsutism
  C. Moon facies
  D. Cervicothoracic obesity
  E. Striae
  F. Easy bruisability
  G. Impaired wound healing
II. Problems secondary to abnormalities on salt and water metabolism
  A. Sodium retention
  B. Weight gain (also increased appetite and polyphagia)
  C. Edema
  D. Increased blood pressure
  E. Hypokalemia (muscle weakness)
III. Endocrine/metabolic problems
  A. Unmask latent diabetes
  B. Aggravate manifest diabetes
  C. Potential for adrenal crises with abrupt discontinuation of Rx or stress
IV. Musculoskeletal
  A. Steroid myopathy with muscle weakness
  B. Osteopenia
  C. Compression fractures
  D. Aseptic necrosis of femoral head
V. Gastrointestinal
  A. Vague abdominal pain
  B. Dyspepsia
  C. ? increased likelihood of GI bleeding
  D. Pancreatitis (controversial)
  E. Mask an acute abdomen
VI. Psychiatric
  A. Depression
  B. Euphoria
  C. Insomnia
  D. Irritability
  E. Psychosis
VII. Hematologic
  A. Leukocytosis
  B. Neutrophilia
  C. Lymphocytopenia
VIII. Immunologic-infectious
  A. False negative skin tests
  B. Increased susceptibility to infections
  C. Opportunistic infections
  D. Reactivation of tuberculosis
  E. Impaired cell mediated immunity
IX. Miscellaneous
  A. Premature cataracts

II-39 LATE COMPLICATIONS OF DIABETES MELLITUS

   I. Atherosclerosis
      A. Coronary artery disease
      B. Cerebrovascular disease
      C. Peripheral vascular disease
  II. Retinopathy
      A. Background
      B. Proliferative
 III. Neuropathy
      A. Peripheral polyneuropathy
      B. Mononeuropathy
      C. Radiculopathy
      D. Amyotrophy
      E. Autonomic neuropathy with esophageal dysfunction, delayed
         gastric emptying, diarrhea, constipation, neurogenic bladder,
         impotence and orthostatic hypotension.
  IV. Nephropathy
   V. Cardiomyopathy
  VI. Hypertriglyceridemia
 VII. Hyporeninemic hypoaldosteronism
VIII. Skin and soft tissue problems
      A. Necrobiosis lipoidica diabeticorum
      B. Diabetic dermopathy
      C. Adipose atrophy or hypertrophy
      D. Impaired wound healing
      E. Foot ulcers
  IX. Increased susceptibility to infections
   X. Cataracts
  XI. Nonalcoholic steatohepatitis

CHAPTER III

Gastroenterology

III-1 CLASSIFICATION OF ESOPHAGEAL MOTILITY DISORDERS

I. Primary
   A. Achalasia
   B. Diffuse esophageal spasm
   C. Variants of achalasia and diffuse esophageal spasm
II. Secondary
   A. Collagen disease
      1. Scleroderma
      2. SLE
      3. Raynaud's disease
      4. Dermatomyositis, polymyositis
   B. Physical, chemical, pharmacologic
      1. Vagotomy
      2. Radiation
      3. Chemical: reflux esophagitis
      4. Drugs (atropine, belladonna alkaloids, Ca++ channel blockers)
   C. Neurologic disease
      1. Cerebrovascular disease
      2. Pseudobulbar palsy
      3. Multiple sclerosis
      4. Amyotrophic lateral sclerosis
      5. Bulbar poliomyelitis
      6. Parkinsonism
   D. Muscle disease
      1. Myotonic dystrophy
      2. Muscular dystrophy
      3. Myasthenia gravis (motor end-plate)
   E. Infection
      1. Chagas' disease *(Trypanosoma cruzi)*
      2. Diphtheria
      3. Tetanus
   F. Metabolic
      1. Diabetes
      2. Alcoholism
      3. Thyrotoxicosis
      4. Myxedema
   G. Miscellaneous
      1. Idiopathic intestinal pseudo-obstruction
      2. Amyloidosis

From Greenberger NJ: *Gastrointestinal disorders: A pathophysiological approach,* ed 4, Chicago, 1989, Year Book Medical Publishers, p. 32.

III-2 ACHALASIA

I. Pathophysiology
  A. Denervation: neuropathy of achalasia
    1. Absence or degeneration of esophageal myenteric ganglion cells
    2. Vagus nerve electron-microscopic alerations: break in continuity of axon-Schwann membranes; swelling of axons; fragmentation of neurofilament; mitochondrial degeneration in axoplasma.
    3. Vagal nucleus: decrease in dorsal motor cells; cytologic distortion of remaining cells.
  B. Functional neuropharmacology
    1. Excessive motor response of the distal esophagus to cholinergic drugs
    2. Supersensitivity of lower esophageal sphincter to gastrin (gastrin acidification) produces reduction in elevated lower esophageal tone to baseline
    3. Other factors: emotional stress, heredity
II. Clinical features
  A. Symptoms: dysphagia for liquids and solids; odynophagia occasionally; regurgitation; tracheobronchial aspiration with pulmonary changes
  B. Signs: weight loss; halitosis; occasionally signs of pulmonary inflammation
III. Diagnosis
  A. Radiography: esophageal dilatation; distal esophagus terminates in a "beak"; aperistalsis; stasis
  B. Esophageal manometry; upper sphincter normal; aperistalsis in body of esophagus; failure of lower esophageal sphincter to relax completely; elevated lower esophageal sphincter resting pressure; hypersensitivity of lower esophageal sphincter to cholinergic drugs
  C. Esophagoscopy: exclude carcinoma, benign stricture; esophageal dilatation; esophagitis
IV. Treatment
  A. Brusque dilatation: forceful dilatation of inferior sphincter with pneumatic or hydrostatic balloon dilator; satisfactory results in 60% to 75%
  B. Surgical therapy: distal esophageal myotomy; satisfactory results in 80%
  C. Botulinum toxin: satisfactory results in 65%; treatments need to be repeated every 6-12 months.

From Greenberger, NJ: N.J., *Gastrointestinal disorders: A pathophysiological approach*, ed 4, Chicago, 1989, Year Book Medical Publishers, p. 33.

III-3   CONDITIONS ASSOCIATED WITH HYPERGASTRINEMIA AND DIAGNOSIS OF ZOLLINGER-ELLISON SYNDROME (ZES)

I. Conditions associated with hypergastrinemia
   A. With acid hypersecretion
      1. Gastrinoma (ZES)
      2. Antral G-cell hyperplasia
      3. Isolated retained gastric antrum
      4. Massive small intestine resection
      5. Hyperparathyroidism
      6. Pyloric outlet obstruction
   B. With variable acid secretion
      1. Hyperthyroidism
      2. Atrophic gastritis
      3. Gastric carcinoma
      4. After vagotomy and pyloroplasty
II. Serum gastrin levels in ZES
   A. >1000 pg/ml with $\uparrow$ [H+] secretion–virtually diagnostic of ZES
   B. 500-1000 pg/ml–strongly suggestive of ZES
   C. 200-500 pg/ml–equivocal; 40% of patients with ZES have a gastrin level in this range
III. Provocative test for ZES
   A. Secretin injection (2 units/kg/IV)→ $\uparrow$ in serum gastrin >200 pg/ml (positive in 90% to 95% of ZES patients)
IV. Somatostatin receptor scintigraphy (SRS) most sensitive imaging method for diagnosing ZES

From Greenberger NJ: *Gastrointestinal disorders: A pathophysiological approach,* ed 4, Chicago, 1989, Year Book Medical Publishers, p. 98.

III-4   DIFFERENTIAL DIAGNOSIS OF REFRACTORY DUODENAL ULCERATION

I. Causes of refractory duodenal ulceration (defined as persistence of ulceration)
   A. Noncompliance
   B. Truly intractable duodenal ulceration
   C. Smoking
   D. *Helicobacter pylori** (failure to eradicate)
   E. Continued use of aspirin and NSAIDs
   F. Gastric acid hypersecretion
      1. Zollinger-Ellison syndrome
      2. Antral G-cell hyperplasia/hyperfunction
      3. Systemic mastocytosis
   G. Pyloric outlet obstruction (incomplete)
   H. Other causes of duodenal ulceration
      1. Crohn's disease
      2. Lymphoma
      3. Primary (duodenal) or secondary (pancreatic) carcinoma
      4. Tuberculosis
II. Causes of postoperative recurrent ulceration
   A. Incomplete vagotomy
   B. ZES
   C. Antral G-cell hyperplasia/hyperfunction
   D. Adjacent nonabsorbable suture
   E. Retained antrum syndrome
   F. Obstruction/delayed gastric emptying
   G. Ulcerogenic drugs

*Especially important in recurrence of duodenal ulcers.

III-5 DELAYED GASTRIC EMPTYING

I. Gastric retention due to pyloric outlet obstruction
    A. Chronic duodenal ulcer diseases
    B. Idiopathic hypertrophic pyloric stenosis
    C. Crohn's disease of the stomach and/or duodenum
    D. Eosinophilic gastroenteritis
    E. Carcinoma of the stomach
    F. Carcinoma of the duodenum or pancreas

II. Acute gastric retention due to mechanical obstruction
    A. Pain
        1. Renal colic
        2. Biliary colic
        3. Recent surgery
    B. Trauma
        1. Retroperitoneal hematoma
        2. Ruptured spleen
        3. Urinary tract injury
    C. Inflammation and infection
        1. Pancreatitis
        2. Peritonitis
        3. Appendicitis
        4. Sepsis
        5. Acute viral gastroenteritis
    D. Immobilization
        1. Body plaster casts
        2. Paraplegia
        3. Postoperative states
    E. Acute gastric retention due to metabolic and electrolyte abnormalities
        1. Diabetic ketoacidosis
        2. Alcoholic ketoacidosis
        3. Myxedema
        4. Acute porphyria
        5. Hepatic coma
        6. Hypokalemia
        7. Hypocalcemia
        8. Hypercalcemia

III. Chronic gastric retention
    A. Neural and smooth muscle disorders
        1. Bulbar poliomyelitis
        2. Brain tumor
        3. Demyelinating diseases (multiple sclerosis)
        4. Vagotomy usually with prior gastric surgery
        5. Scleroderma
        6. Idiopathic intestinal pseudo-obstruction

Continued

III-5   DELAYED GASTRIC EMPTYING—*cont'd*

  B. Metabolic disorders
     1. Diabetes mellitus (vagal neuropathy may be present)
     2. Myxedema
     3. Drugs
       a. Anticholinergics
       b. Opiates (morphine, codeine, etc.)
       c. Ganglionic blockers
       d. Aluminum-containing antacids
       e. Pectin and ?psyllium hydrophilic mucilloids
     4. Psychiatric disease
       a. Anorexia nervosa
     5. Idiopathic
       a. Antecedent viral illnesses

From Greenberger NJ: *Gastrointestinal disorders: A pathophysiological approach,* ed 4, Chicago, 1989, Year Book Medical Publishers, p. 113.

III-6   DIAGNOSIS OF ANOREXIA NERVOSA

   I. Age of onset before 25 yr
  II. Anorexia with weight loss > 25% of original body weight
 III. Distorted, implacable attitude toward eating, food, or weight that overrides hunger, admonitions, reassurance, and threats, e.g.:
    A. Denial of illness with failure to recognize nutritional needs
    B. Enjoyment in losing weight
    C. Desired body image of extreme thinness with evidence that it is rewarding to achieve and maintain this state
    D. Unusual hoarding or handling of food
 IV. No known medical illness to account for anorexia and weight loss
  V. No other psychiatric disorder
 VI. At least two of the following:
    A. Amenorrhea
    B. Lanugo
    C. Bradycardia
    D. Overactivity
    E. Bulimia
    F. Vomiting (may be self-induced)

From Drossman D et al: *Gastroenterology* 77:1117, 1979.

III-7   CLASSIFICATION OF THE MALABSORPTION SYNDROMES

I. Inadequate digestion
   A. Postgastrectomy steatorrhea*
   B. Deficiency or inactivation of pancreatic lipase
      1. Exocrine pancreatic insufficiency
         a. Chronic pancreatitis
         b. Pancreatic carcinoma
         c. Cystic fibrosis
         d. Pancreatic resection
      2. Ulcerogenic tumor of the pancreas (Zollinger-Ellison syndrome*)
II. Reduced intestinal bile salt concentration (with impaired formation of micellar lipid)
   A. Liver disease
      1. Parenchymal liver disease
      2. Cholestasis (intrahepatic or extrahepatic)
   B. Abnormal bacterial proliferation in the small bowel
      1. Afferent loop stasis
      2. Strictures
      3. Fistulas
      4. Blind loops
      5. Multiple diverticula of the small bowel
      6. Hypomotility states (diabetes, scleroderma); intestinal pseudo-obstruction
   C. Interrupted enterohepatic circulation of bile salts
      1. Ileal resection
      2. Ileal inflammatory disease (regional ileitis)
   D. Drug-induced (by sequestration or precipitation of bile salts)
      1. Neomycin
      2. Calcium carbonate
      3. Cholestyramine
III. Inadequate absorptive surface
   A. Intestinal resection or bypass
      1. Mesenteric vascular disease with massive intestinal resection
      2. Regional enteritis with multiple bowel resection
      3. Jejunoileal bypass
   B. Gastroileostomy

Continued

III-7 CLASSIFICATION OF THE MALABSORPTION SYNDROMES—*cont'd*

IV. Lymphatic obstruction
- A. Intestinal lymphangiectasia
- B. Whipple's disease*
- C. Lymphoma*
- D. Kohlmeier-Degos (primary progressive arterial occlusive disease)*

V. Cardiovasular disorders
- A. Constrictive pericarditis
- B. Congestive heart failure
- C. Mesenteric vascular insufficiency
- D. Collagen vascular disease

VI. Endocrine and metabolic disorders
- A. Diabetes mellitus
- B. Hypoparathyroidism
- C. Adrenal insufficiency
- D. Hyperthyroidism
- E. Ulcerogenic tumor of the pancreas (Zollinger-Ellison syndrome*)
- F. Carcinoid syndrome

VII. Primary mucosal absorptive defects
- A. Inflammatory or infiltrative disorders
  1. Regional enteritis*
  2. Amyloidosis
  3. Scleroderma*
  4. Lymphoma*
  5. Eosinophilic enteritis
  6. Tropical sprue
  7. Infectious enteritis (e.g., salmonellosis)
  8. Mucosal lesions associated with intestinal bacterial growth
- B. Biochemical or genetic abnormalities
  1. Celiac sprue
  2. Abetalipoproteinemia
  3. Hartnup disease
  4. Cystinuria
  5. Hypogammaglobulinemia

*Multiple mechanisms responsible for malabsorption.

III-8   DIAGNOSIS OF CELIAC SPRUE

  I. Evidence of malabsorption
   A. Isolated or generalized
    1. ↓ D-xylose, steatorrhea, ↓ Ca++, Fe++, albumin, choles-
      terol, carotenes, B_{12} absorption, ↑ protime, etc.
 II. Abnormal small bowel mucosal biopsy
III. Improvement (clinical, laboratory tests, intestinal histology) with
    gluten-free diet
 IV. Exacerbation of symptoms, diarrhea, and steatorrhea with gluten
    challenge
   A. Should be used only in equivocal cases
  V. Positive antiendomysial antibody >90% cases

III-9   CELIAC SPRUE—FAILURE TO RESPOND
TO GLUTEN-FREE DIET

   I. Incorrect diagnosis
  II. Nonadherence to gluten-free diet
 III. Unsuspected concurrent disease such as pancreatic insufficiency
 IV. Development of intestinal lymphoma
  V. Development of diffuse intestinal ulceration
 VI. Presence of nongranulomatous ulcerative jejunoileitis
VII. Presence of diffuse collagen deposits, i.e., "collagenous sprue"
VIII. Presence of lymphocytic (microscopic) colitis

III-10   CONDITIONS ASSOCIATED WITH BACTERIAL
OVERGROWTH

   I. Billroth II subtotal gastrectomy with afferent loop stasis
  II. Blind loops
 III. Multiple small bowel diverticula
 IV. Hypomotility states (diabetes, scleroderma, intestinal pseudo-
    obstruction)
  V. Incomplete small bowel obstruction
 VI. Gastric achlorhydria (pernicious anemia)
VII. Strictures (regional enteritis, radiation injury)
VIII. Fistulas (regional enteritis)

III-11   DIAGNOSIS OF "BACTERIAL OVERGROWTH" SYNDROME

 *I. Steatorrhea–usually moderate (15-30 gm/day)
 II. D-xylose–can be normal or abnormal
 III. Small bowel biopsy–can be normal or abnormal
 *IV. Vitamin B_{12} absorption with IF
 *V. (+) Small bowel culture
    A. Usually $>10^7$ organisms/ml
    B. Polymicrobial (*E. coli,* bacteroides, enterococci, anaerobic lactobacilli)
 VI. Abnormal breath tests (lactulose, ^{14}C-xylose, and so on)

*Correction of #1, 4, and 5 with antibiotic therapy.

III-12   CLINICAL FEATURES OF ZINC DEFICIENCY

 I. Skin
    A. Acrodermatitis enteropathica
    B. Alopecia
    C. Poor wound healing
 II. Neuropsychiatric
    A. Depression
    B. Irritability
    C. Lack of concentration
    D. Tremor
 III. Eyes
    A. Night blindness
 IV. Gastrointestinal
    A. Anorexia
    B. Impaired taste
    C. Diarrhea
 V. Pancreatic insufficiency
    A. Endocrine
    B. Hypogonadism
    C. Dwarfism in children
    D. Insulin hypersensitivity

From Tasman-Jones C. In Stollerman G (ed): *Advances in internal medicine,* vol 26, Chicago, 1980, Year Book Medical Publishers, p. 105.

III-13   DIFFERENTIAL DIAGNOSIS OF REGIONAL ENTERITIS

  I. Infectious enteritis (bacterial, fungal, protozoal)
      A. Must exclude amebiasis, campylobacter, yersinia, chlamydia
 II. Tuberculous enteritis
III. Lymphoma
 IV. Carcinoid tumor
  V. Carcinoma
 VI. Intestinal lymphangiectasia
VII. Ischemic small bowel disease with/without segmental infarcts
      A. Connective tissue disease with vasculitis (PN, SLE)
      B. Atherosclerotic/embolic disease
VIII. Malabsorptive disorders with primary gut involvement
      A. Celiac sprue
      B. Amyloidosis
      C. Whipple's disease
 IX. Nongranulomatous ulcerative jejunoileitis
  X. Eosinophilic gastroenteritis
 XI. Nonsteroidal antiinflammatory drugs (NSAIDs)

III-14 FEATURES DIFFERENTIATING IDIOPATHIC ULCERATIVE COLITIS FROM GRANULOMATOUS COLITIS*

Features	Ulcerative colitis	Granulomatous colitis
I. CLINICAL FEATURES		
Diarrhea	+ + + +	+ + +
Hematochezia	+ + + +	+ +
Abdominal tenderness	+ +	+ + +
Abdominal mass	0	+ + to + + +
Toxic megacolon	+	+
Perforation	+	+
Fistulas		
Perianal, perineal	0	+ +
Enteroenteric	0	+
II. ENDOSCOPIC FEATURES (sigmoidoscopy, colonoscopy)		
Rectal involvement	+ + + +	+ +
Diffuse, continuous disease	+ + + +	+
Friability, purulence	+ + + to + + +	+
Aphthous, linear ulcers	0	+ + + to + + + +
Cobblestoning	0	+ + to + + +
Pseudopolyps	+ +	+
III. RADIOLOGIC FEATURES		
Continuous disease	+ + + +	0 to +
Associated ileal disease	0	+ +
Strictures	0	+ to + +
Fistulas	0	+ to + +
Asymmetric wall involvement	0	+ + to + + +
Fissures	0	+ to + +
IV. PATHOLOGIC FEATURES		
Granulomas	0	+ + + to + + + +
Transmural inflammation	0 to +	+ + + to + + + +
Crypt abscess	+ + +	+ to + +
Skip areas of involvement	0	+ + +
Linear, aphthous ulcers	0	+ + + to + + + +

*Key: 0 = never or rarely; + = <25%; + + = 25-50%; + + + = 50-75%; + + + + = >75%.
From Greenberger NJ: *Gastrointestinal disorders: A pathophysiological approach,* ed 4, Chicago, 1989, Year Book Medical Publishers, p. 226.

III-15   SYSTEMIC MANIFESTATIONS OF ULCERATIVE COLITIS (UC) AND REGIONAL ENTERITIS (RE)

	UC	RE
I. Skin		
A. Erythema nodosum	+	+
B. Pyoderma gangrenosum	+	+
C. Ulcerating erythematous plaques	+	+
II. Eyes		
A. Uveitis	+	+
III. Mouth		
A. Aphthous ulcers, cheilitis	±	+
IV. Esophagus		
A. Ulceration	+	+
V. Stomach and duodenum		
A. Pyloric outlet obstruction	—	+
VI. Small bowel		
A. Malabsorption	—	+
B. Lactose intolerance	+	+
VII. Liver		
A. Steatosis	+	+
B. Cirrhosis	+	+
C. Chronic active liver disease	+	+
D. Granulomas	—	+
VIII. Gallbladder and biliary tree		
A. Cholelithiasis	—	+
B. Sclerosing cholangitis	+	rarely present
C. Bile duct carcinoma	+	—
IX. Renal disease		
A. Obstructive hydronephrosis	—	+
B. Nephrolithiasis	+(urate)	+(oxalate)
X. Anemia		
A. Blood loss	+	+
B. Hemolysis	+	+
C. Folate depletion (sulfasalazine)	+	+
D. Chronic illness	+	+
XI. Thrombocytosis	+	+
XII. Pulmonary		
A. Fibrosing alveolitis	+	—
B. Pulmonary vasculitis	+	—
XIII. Pancreatitis		
A. Ductal obstruction	—	+
B. Drugs (azathioprine, sulfasalazine, steroids)	+	+
XIV. Vulva (Crohn's disease)	—	+
XV. Joints		
A. Arthritis	+	+

III-16   CLASSIFICATION, DIAGNOSIS, AND MANAGEMENT OF CHRONIC DIARRHEAL DISORDERS

Cause	Examples	Key elements in diagnosis	Treatment
1. Iatrogenic dietary factors	Excess tea, coffee, cola beverages, simple sugars	Careful history taking	Appropriate dietary modifications
2. Infectious enteritis	Amebiasis Giardiasis	Demonstrate leukocytes in stool Identify trophozoites or cysts in stool and duodenal aspirate (giardiasis)	Amebiasis—metronidazole diodoquin antibiotics Giardiasis—metronidazole
3. Inflammatory bowel disease	Ulcerative colitis Regional enteritis	History: Diarrhea, abdominal pain, rectal bleeding Sigmoidoscopy, barium enema, UGI, and small bowel series	Sulfasalazine Corticosteroids
4. Irritable bowel syndrome	See Table III-16	See Table III-17 Antispasmodics	Dietary modifications
5. Incontinence	Diabetes Rectal surgery Radiation proctitis	History	Depends on cause
6. Idiopathic secretory		Stool output >1.0 L/24 hr, No ↓ stool volume with fasting, Stool osmolality gap 40mOsm/kg	
7. Lactose intolerance	Milk intolerance	Milk → abdominal pain, diarrhea, gas, bloating. Cessation of milk drinking → amelioration of symptoms Lactose load (1 gm/kg) → exacerbation of symptoms and breath H_2 fails to rise	Discontinue milk

Cause	Examples	Key elements in diagnosis	Treatment
8. Laxative abuse		Add a few drops of NaOH to stool. Because most laxatives contain phenolphthalein, the stool will turn red.	Discontinue laxative
9. Drug-induced	Antacids, antibiotics (clindamycin, ampicillin, penicillin), NSAIDs, colchicine, lactulose, sorbitol	Careful history taking and review of medication.	Discontinue offending drug
10. Diverticular and pre-diverticular disease		History: intermittent symptoms PE: Palpable LF. colon Barium enema: diverticulosis and/or muscle hypertrophy	High fiber diet. Avoid: corn, nuts, peanuts, kernel-containing foods.
11. Malabsorptive disease	Pancreatic insufficiency Regional enteritis Short bowel Bacterial overgrowth	UGI plus small bowel x-rays; tests of intestinal absorptive function: D-xylose, stool fat, Schilling test, serum carotenes, calcium, albumin, cholesterol, iron, prothrombin time	Appropriate for the underlying disorder
12. Metabolic	Diabetes mellitus Hyperthyroidism Adrenal insufficiency	Abnormal blood glucose levels $\uparrow T_4$, $\downarrow$ TSH, $\uparrow$ RAI uptake $\downarrow$ plasma cortisol, $\downarrow$ response to synthetic ACTH	Appropriate for the underlying disorder
13. Mechanical	Fecal impaction	Rectal examination	Remove impaction

Continued

III-16 CLASSIFICATION, DIAGNOSIS, AND MANAGEMENT OF CHRONIC DIARRHEAL DISORDERS—*cont'd*

Cause	Examples	Key elements in diagnosis	Treatment
14. Neoplastic	Carcinoma of the pancreas Carcinoid syndrome Villous adenoma Medullary carcinoma of the thyroid Tumors producing V.I.P. (vasoactive intestinal peptide) Gastrinoma	Suspect the diagnosis	Surgical
15. Postoperative history	Gastric surgery Intestinal resection (especially ileum) Short bowel syndrome		

III-17   DIAGNOSIS OF IRRITABLE BOWEL SYNDROME

I. Criteria useful in establishing the diagnosis
   A. Usual criteria
      1. Symptoms: abdominal pain, diarrhea, alternating diarrhea and constipation, relief of abdominal pain with defecation, feeling of incomplete evacuation with defecation, absence of nocturnal symptoms
      2. Absence of systemic symptoms: anorexia, weight loss, fever, and signs, i.e., anemia
      3. No hematochezia, melena, or occult blood in stool
      4. Normal sigmoidoscopy
      5. Normal barium enema
   B. Additional criteria if symptoms persist
      1. Normal stool weight (24 hr stool weight <300 gm)
      2. No steatorrhea or evidence of malabsorption
      3. Normal upper gastrointestinal tract and small bowel x-ray films
II. Differential diagnosis
   A. Lactose intolerance
   B. Other disaccharidase deficiencies, i.e., sucrose-isomaltose intolerance
   C. Subclinical carbohydrate malabsorption
   D. Diverticular and "prediverticular disease"
   E. Drug-induced diarrhea
   F. Idiopathic bile acid malabsorption
   G. Inadvertent dietary indiscretion (excess caffeine, tea, cola beverages, and so on)
   H. Irritable bowel disorder not associated with an underlying disorder
   I. Motility disorders small bowel or colon (incompletely defined)

III-18 RISK FACTORS FOR DEVELOPING COLON CANCER

I. Age >40 years
II. Family history of colon cancer
III. Prior colon carcinoma
IV. Familial polyposis
V. Gardner's syndrome
VI. Villous adenoma
VII. Colonic polyps with advanced features
    A. >1.0 cm
    B. Villous or tubulovillous histology
VIII. Idiopathic ulcerative colitis
IX. Granulomatous colitis (Crohn's disease)
X. Prior breast or female genital tract cancer
XI. Asbestosis
XII. Diet rich in beef and lipid
XIII. Acromegaly (data incomplete)
XIV. Peutz-Jeghers syndrome
XV. Postcholecystectomy (controversial)

From Greenberger NJ: *Gastrointestinal disorders: A pathophysiological approach,* ed 4. Chicago, 1989, Year Book Medical Publishers, p. 240.

III-19 DIAGNOSIS OF CHRONIC ALCOHOLISM

I. Evidence of alcohol withdrawal syndromes
    A. Tremulousness
    B. Alcoholic hallucinosis
    C. Withdrawal seizures or "rum fits"
    D. Delirium tremens
II. Evidence of tolerance to alcohol
    A. Ingestion of 1 fifth or more of whiskey per day
    B. No gross evidence of intoxication with blood alcohol level > 150 mg/100 ml
    C. Random blood alcohol level > 300 mg/100 ml
    D. Accelerated clearance of blood alcohol (> 25 mg/100 ml per hour)
III. Psychosociologic factors
    A. Continued ingestion of alcohol despite strong contraindication to do so:
        1. Threatened loss of job
        2. Threatened loss of spouse and/or family
        3. Medical contraindication known to patient
    B. Admission of inability to discontinue use of alcohol

Continued

III-19 DIAGNOSIS OF CHRONIC ALCOHOLISM—*cont'd*

IV. Presence of alcohol-associated disorders
   A. Erosive gastritis with upper gastrointestinal bleeding
   B. Pancreatitis, acute and chronic, in the absence of cholelithiasis
   C. Alcoholic liver disease (fatty liver, alcoholic hepatitis, cirrhosis)
   D. Alcoholic diseases of the nervous system
      1. Peripheral neuropathy
      2. Cerebellar degeneration
      3. Wernicke-Korsakoff syndrome
      4. Beriberi
      5. Alcoholic myopathy
      6. Alcoholic cardiomyopathy
V. "CAGE" criteria
   A. C = Concerned about drinking
   B. A = Annoyed about questions on drinking
   C. G = Guilty about drinking
   D. E = Eye opener, i.e., morning drink needed

III-20 SPECTRUM OF ALCOHOLIC LIVER DISEASE

I. Alcoholic fatty liver
   A. Clear cytoplasmic vacuoles
   B. Eccentrically placed cell nuclei
II. Alcoholic hepatitis
   A. Polymorphonuclear infiltration
   B. Alcoholic hyaline
   C. Central hyaline necrosis and sclerosis of central vein
   D. Fat and/or fibrosis may be present
III. Alcoholic cirrhosis
   A. Distortion of lobular architecture
   B. Fibrous septa involving portal and central zones
IV. Secondary changes
   A. Cholestasis
   B. Bile duct proliferation
   C. Siderosis
   D. Fat

III-21 CLINICAL AND HISTOLOGIC FEATURES OF ALCOHOLIC HEPATITIS

I. Clinical features
   A. General considerations: Spectrum of clinical findings ranging from asymptomatic to florid decompensated liver disease with hepatosplenomegaly, jaundice, ascites, azotemia, and encephalopathy
   B. Symptoms: Anorexia, weakness, abdominal pain, weight loss, fever
   C. Signs: Jaundice, peripheral stigmata of chronic liver disease, hepatomegaly, splenomegaly, ascites, edema, signs of hepatic encephalopathy
   D. Laboratory data: ↑ MCV, ↑ WBC, ↑ SGOT, ↑ SGOT:SGPT (AST:ALT) > 3:1, ↑ bilirubin, ↓ albumin, prolonged prothrombin time
   E. Histologic features of alcoholic hepatitis
      1. Absolute criteria
         a. Hepatocellular necrosis
         b. Polymorphonuclear infiltration of the liver
      2. Generally accepted criteria
         a. Mallory alcoholic hyaline
      3. Often present but not required for the diagnosis
         a. Fatty infiltration of the liver
         b. Fibrosis
         c. Cirrhosis
   F. Diagnosis of alcoholic hepatitis
      1. History of excessive alcohol intake
      2. Liver biopsy showing changes of alcoholic hepatitis
      3. Lab: ↑ MCV, ↑ SGOT, ↑ GGTP, ↑ SGOT:SGPT ratio
   G. Indicators of a bad prognosis
      1. Serum bilirubin > 20 mg/dl
      2. BUN > 25 mg/dl without obvious cause
      3. Hepatic encephalopathy
      4. Prothrombin time prolonged > 6 seconds compared to controls

III-22   HEPATITIS A

I. General considerations
  A. Short incubation period (14-24 days)
  B. Fecal-oral transmission (epidemics with contaminated water)
  C. Virus present in stools from incubation period to onset of clinical illness
  D. Triad of headache, fever, myalgias favors hepatitis A over hepatitis B
  E. Maximum period of infectivity 2 weeks after onset of clinical illness
  F. Frequently anicteric
  G. Does not result in chronic liver disease
  H. Infection confers immunity
II. Immunologic considerations
  A. Hepatitis A antigen (HA Ag) circulates transiently at low titers
  B. HA Ag cleared rapidly from stool
  C. HA Ag detection in serum and stool not feasible clinically
  D. HA Ab rises rapidly, peaks after 2-3 months, persists
  *E. HA Ab in acute phase is IgM; later ($\geq$4 months) is IgG
  F. HA Ab present in majority of adults ($>$ 50% at age $>$ 60)
  G. Conventional immune serum globulin *modifies* the disease

*IgM antibody persists for $>$ 120 days in $>$ 10% of patients.

From Greenberger NJ: *Gastrointestinal disorders: A pathophysiological approach,* ed 4, Chicago, 1989, Year Book Medical Publishers, p. 317.

III-23 HEPATITIS C

I. General information
   A. Reservoir of 3.5 million cases in the United States
   B. Estimated 50,000-100,000 new cases/year with second and third generation screening tests
   C. Incubation period 6 to 14 weeks (mean, 7 to 8)
   D. Hepatitis C antigen demonstrable in liver

II. Role of hepatitis C in liver disease
   A. Acute hepatitis
   B. Chronic hepatitis (70% to 75% of population with acute hepatitis C)
   C. Cirrhosis (20% to 25% of patients with acute hepatitis C)
   D. Alcoholic liver disease (hepatitis C may potentiate development)
   E. Hepatocellular carcinoma (25% to 60% test hepatitis C virus (HCV) positive)

III. Epidemiologic settings
   A. Transfusion associated (acute as well as remote)
   B. Parenteral drug abuse
   C. Transplant patients
   D. Multiply transfused hemophiliacs
   E. Hemodialysis patients
   F. Prisoners; institutionalized individuals
   G. Health care workers
   H. Tattoos, shared razors, shared toothbrushes
   I. High risk sexual behavior (promiscuity, sex with prostitute, sexually transmitted disease)
   J. Intranasal cocaine use
   K. Unknown risk factors identified (30%)

IV. Clinical factors
   A. Patient often asymptomatic and frequently detected by elevated serum aminotransferase
   B. Histologic changes of chronic hepatitis/cirrhosis may not correlate with physical findings or liver test abnormalities.
   C. Third generation test for hepatitis C virus (HCV-antibody) positive in 90% patients with acute hepatitis C
   D. Evidence of hepatitis C infection (either HCV-antibody or HCV-RNA) persists for many years after infection
   E. Disease can be latent for many years
   F. Positive HCV-RNA associated with abnormal liver histology

V. Treatment
   A. Interferon alpha 2B given for 6 to 12 months results in clinical response in 50% to 65% of patients, half of whom relapse within 6 months after discontinuation of therapy

III-24   HEPATITIS B

Epidemiologic considerations

Long incubation period (50-180 days)
Transmitted by parenteral and nonparenteral routes
HB_sAg: spheres, tubules, Dane particles
Spheres and tubules represent viral surface coat material made in infected hepatocytes
Dane particle contains inner core antigen (HB_cAg) and outer shell (HB_sAg) and represents complete virion
HB_sAg detected in blood, saliva, urine, semen, breast milk, bile
Sexual partners, homosexuals, and newborn infants have high rate of infection

Immunologic considerations

Antigen	Significance	Antibody	Significance
HB_sAg	Hepatitis B infection	Anti-HB_s (HB_sAb)	Denotes prior hepatitis B infection and usually immunity
HB_cAg	Hepatitis B infection	Anti-HB_o (HB_cAb)	Recent or ongoing infection HB_sAg carriers—high titers
DNA polymerase	High infectivity; viral replication		
HB_eAg	Suggests high infectivity; associated with active disease	Anti-HB_C (HB_CAb)	Suggests limited/no disease activity and low-grade infectivity
Delta antigen	Infection with Delta agent	Delta antibody	Accelerated course of cronic hepatitis; increased risk of fulminant hepatitis

Continued

III-24   HEPATITIS B—*cont'd*

Diagnosis of hepatitis B (HBV) infection

HB_sAg positive in 75-85% of HBV infections
Reasons:
   HBV present but below detectable concentrations
   HBV cleared, no HB_sAb (serologic window)
   DX in HB_sAg negative patients established by demonstrating HB_sAb
   (+)HB_sAg or other HBV markers in 30-40% chronic active liver disease patients

Spectrum of responses in hepatitis B infections

Acute icteric hepatitis
   Serum bilirubin > 3.0 mg/dl
   Serum transaminases > 100 on > 2 occasions 4 days apart
Acute anicteric hepatitis
   Serum bilirubin < 3.0 mg/dl
   Serum transaminases > 100 on > 2 occasions 4 days apart
Seroconversion with HB_sAg positivity
   $HB_sAg \rightarrow HB_sAb$
Seroconversion without HB_sAg positivity
   HB_sAb (−) $\rightarrow HB_sAb$ (+)

Interpretation of serological abnormalities in hepatitis B infection

	Tests				Interpretations
	HBsAg	HBcAb	HBsAb		
1.	+	−	−	1. a.	Acute viral hepatitis
2.	+	+	−	2. a.	Acute viral hepatitis
				b.	Chronic active hepatitis or
					Chronic persistent hepatitis
				c.	Chronic carrier state
3.	−	+	−	3. a.	Acute viral hepatitis (in window phase)
				b.	Remote B viral infection
4.	−	+	+	4. a.	Remote B viral infection
				b.	Chronic hepatitis in immunosuppressed patient (HBsAb titer is usually low)
				c.	Subclinical infection
5.	−	−	+	5. a.	Remote B viral infection
				b.	Immunization response
6.	+	−	+	6. a.	Remote and recent B viral infection

From Greenberger NJ: *Gastrointestinal disorders: A pathophysiological approach*, ed 4, Chicago, 1989, Year Book Medical Publishers, pp. 318-319.

III-25 ETIOLOGY AND DIAGNOSIS OF CHRONIC HEPATITIS

I. Causes of chronic hepatitis
  A. Autoimmune
  B. Viral hepatitis, type B
  C. Viral hepatitis, type C
  D. Drugs
    1. Alpha-methyldopa*
    2. Aspirin (especially in patients with rheumatoid arthritis)
    3. Acetaminophen
    4. Allopurinol
    5. Halothane
    6. Isoniaxid*
    7. Nitrofurantoin*
    8. Oxyphenisatin
    9. Propylthiouracil
    10. Sulfonamides
    11. Interferon Alpha 2B
  E. Miscellaneous
    1. Wilson's disease
    2. Alpha-1 antitrypsin disease
    3. Alcohol
II. Diagnosis of chronic hepatitis†
  A. Persistence of symptoms and signs of liver disease for >6 months
  B. Persistence of abnormal liver tests for >6 months
    1. ↑ Aminotransferase
    2. ↑ Gammaglobulins
  C. Abnormal hepatic histology
    1. Chronic hepatitis without cirrhosis
      a. Periportal and piecemeal necrosis with portal zone expansion and rosette formation
      b. Multilobular necrosis
      c. Bridging (confluent) hepatic necrosis
      d. Periportal plus piecemeal necrosis
    2. Chronic hepatitis with cirrhosis

*Most important.
†Demonstration of ongoing activity for at least 6 months emphasizes the unresolving nature of the process and is desirable for establishing the diagnosis. However, the onset of illness may be difficult to estimate. Thus patients with disease of less than 6 months duration may develop hypoalbuminemia, hypergammaglobulinemia, and ascites; and present simulating acute hepatitis.

III-26 PRIMARY BILIARY CIRRHOSIS

I. Diagnosis
   A. Hepatomegaly
   B. ↑ Serum alkaline phosphatase
   C. (+) test for antimitochondrial antibody
   D. ↑ IgM levels
   E. ↑ Serum cholesterol
   F. Compatible histologic changes on liver biopsy
   G. Exclusion of extrahepatic obstruction

II. Natural history of primary biliary cirrhosis
   A. Hepatomegaly
   B. Pruritus
   C. Increased pigmentation
   D. Hyperbilirubinemia
   E. Xanthomata
   F. Splenomegaly
   G. Ascites
   H. GI bleeding
   I. Encephalopathy

Appearance of clinical features as course of the disease progresses

III. Liver transplantation

III-27   COMMON PRECIPITATING CAUSES OF HEPATIC ENCEPHALOPATHY

Causes	Possible mechanisms leading to coma
I. Azotemia (spontaneous or induced diuresis)	↑ BUN leads to ↑ endogenous NH_3 production; direct suppressive effect on brain from uremia
II. Sedatives, tranquilizers, anesthetics	Direct depressive effect on brain; impaired metabolism of sedative drugs with hepatic parenchymal cell failure
III. Gastrointestinal hemorrhage	Provides substrate for increased NH_3 production (100 ml blood = 15-20 gm protein)
	Shock and hypoxia
	Hypovolemia → impaired cerebral, hepatic, and renal function
	Azotemia can lead to further ↑ in blood NH_3 due to load of NH_3 from transfused blood (Storage at 4° C: 1 day = 170 mg/100 ml; 4 days = 330; 21 days = 900.)
IV. Diuretics	Induce ↓ K^+ alkalosis
	↓ K^+ leads to ↑ renal output NH_3 across blood-brain barrier
	Vigorous diuresis can result in hypovolemia and impaired cardiac, cerebral, hepatic, and renal function, the latter resulting in azotemia; azotemia ↑ endogenous NH_3 production
V. Metabolic alkalosis	Favors transfer of nonionized NH_3 across blood-brain barrier
VI. Increased dietary protein intake	Provides substrate for increased NH_3 production
VII. Infection	↑ Tissue catabolism leading to ↑ endogenous NH_3 load
	Dehydration and impaired renal function
	Hypoxia, hypotension, hyperthermia may potentiate NH_3 toxicity
VIII. Constipation	Intestinal production and absorption of NH_3 and other nitrogenous products
IX. Hepatic injury	Superimposed viral or toxic parenchymal cell injury may compromise liver function
X. Miscellaneous	NH_4-containing drugs (NH_4Cl)
	Acquired form of renal tubular acidosis (distal type) with inappropriate kaliuresis
	Genetic disorders with specific deficiency of urea cycle enzymes
	Presence of hypoglycemia, hypercarbia, or severe hypoxemia in patients with marginal hepatocellular function
	H. pylori infection (increased urease activity)

III-28   DIFFERENTIAL DIAGNOSIS OF ASCITES

I. Transudative effusions
- A. Cirrhosis*
- B. Congestive heart failure*
- C. Constrictive pericarditis*
- D. Obstruction to the hepatic veins (Budd-Chiari syndrome)*
   1. Associated with tumors (hepatoma, hypernephroma, cancer of the pancreas)
   2. Associated with hematologic disorders (myeloproliferative disease, polycythemia vera, myeloid metaplasia)
- E. Obstruction to the inferior vena cava
- F. Nephrotic syndrome
- G. Viral hepatitis
- H. Meig's syndrome
- I. Myelofibrosis
- J. Spontaneous bacterial perontonitis (BSP)

II. Exudative effusions
- A. Neoplastic diseases involving the peritoneum
   1. Peritoneal carcinomatosis
   2. Lymphomatous disorders
- B. Tuberculous peritonitis
- C. Pancreatitis* (also leading pseudocyst and disrupted main pancreatic duct)
- D. Talc or starch powder peritonitis after surgery
- E. Transected lymphatics after porta-caval shunt surgery
- F. Myxedema
- G. Sarcoidosis
- H. Lymphatic obstruction
   1. Intestinal lymphangiectasia
   2. Lymphomas
- I. Pseudomyxoma peritonei
- J. Struma ovarii
- K. Amyloidosis
- L. Prior abdominal trauma with ruptured lymphatics
- M. Nephrogenic ascites†
- N. Primary bacterial peritonitis (PBP)

III. Disorders simulating ascites
- A. Pancreatic pseudocyst
- B. Hydronephrosis
- C. Ovarian cyst
- D. Mesenteric cyst
- E. Obesity

*Most common disorders.
†Occurs in patients with renal failure on maintenance hemodialysis.
From Greenberger NJ: *Gastrointestinal disorders: A pathological approach,* ed 4, Chicago, 1989, Year Book Medical Publishers, p. 367.

III-29   CONDITIONS CAUSING OR CONTRIBUTING TO POSTOPERATIVE JAUNDICE

I. Increased load of bilirubin pigment
   A. Hemolytic anemia
   B. Resorption of hematomas or hemoperitoneum
   C. Pulmonary infarction
   D. Transfusions: If blood stored >1 week, approximately 10% of red blood cells hemolyzed → extra load of ~7.5 gm hemoglobin. $7.5 \times 35 = {\sim}250$ mg extra bilirubin/unit blood

II. Impaired hepatocellular function
   A. Hepatitis-like picture
      1. Post-transfusion hepatitis
         a. Hepatitis B, hepatitis C (now rare)
         b. Cytomegalovirus, EB virus, adenovirus, ECHO, coxsackie
      2. Hypotension
      3. Halothane anesthesia
      4. Drugs
   B. Intrahepatic cholestasis
      1. Hypotension
      2. Hypoxemia
      3. Sepsis
      4. Drugs
      5. Total parenteral nutrition
   C. Congestive heart failure

III. Extrahepatic biliary tract obstruction
   A. Bile duct injury
   B. Choledocholithiasis

III-30 DIFFERENTIAL DIAGNOSIS OF INTRAHEPATIC CHOLESTASIS*

I. Hepatocellular
   A. Viral hepatitis
   B. Alcoholic hepatitis
   C. Chronic active hepatitis
   D. Alpha-1 antitrypsin deficiency

II. Hepatocanalicular
   A. Drugs (17-alkylated steroids, phenothiazines)
   B. Sepsis
   C. Toxic shock syndrome
   D. Postoperative
   E. Total parenteral nutrition
   F. Neoplasms (Hodgkin's disease, lymphoma, prostatic carcinoma)
   G. Sickle cell anemia
   H. Amyloidosis

III. Ductular
   A. Sarcoidosis
   B. Primary biliary cirrhosis

IV. Ducts
   A. Intrahepatic biliary atresia
   B. Intrahepatic sclerosing cholangitis
   C. Caroli's disease
   D. Cholangiocarcinoma

V. Recurrent cholestasis
   A. Benign recurrent intrahepatic cholestasis
   B. Recurrent jaundice of pregnancy
   C. Dubin-Johnson syndrome

*Classification based on apparent site of hepatic injury.

III-31 DIFFERENTIAL DIAGNOSIS OF IRON STORAGE DISEASE AND CLINICAL FEATURES OF IDIOPATHIC HEMOCHROMATOSIS

	Iron overload in family members	Anemia	Cirrhosis	Transferrin saturation	Serum* ferritin	Desferrioxamine iron excretion
I. Refractory anemias	0	+	0	Normal to ↑	Variable	Variable
II. Laennec's cirrhosis	0	±	+	Normal	Normal to ↑	2-4 mg/24 hr
III. Excess oral iron intake	0	±	0	↑	Normal to ↑	Variable
IV. Transfusion	0	+	0	↑	↑	Variable
V. Idiopathic hemochromatosis†	+	0	±	> 80%	> 1000 ng/ml	>8 mg/24hr
A. Skin pigmentation						
B. Diabetes mellitus						
C. Hepatomegaly, splenomegaly, cirrhosis						
D. Hypogonadism						
E. Cardiomyopathy and congestive heart failure						
F. Adrenal insufficiency						
G. Arthropathy						

+ = present; 0 = absent; ± = may or may not be present.
*Hepatic iron index is more reliable.
†Liver biopsy shows parenchymal distribution of iron deposits.

From Greenberger NJ: *Gastrointestinal disorders: A pathophysiological approach*, ed 4, Chicago, 1989, Year Book Medical Publishers, p. 388.

III-32   COMPARISON OF THE CLINICAL, RADIOLOGIC, AND PATHOLOGIC CHARACTERISTICS OF FOCAL NODULAR HYPERPLASIA AND LIVER CELL ADENOMA

	Focal nodular hyperplasia	Liver cell adenoma
I. Clinical		
Incidence	Uncommon	Rare
Age	All ages	Third, fourth decades
Sex	85% F	Nearly all F
Oral contraceptive use	Occasionally	Nearly always
Clinical presentation	Usually asymptomatic 35% have abdominal mass, abdominal discomfort	Often abdominal emergency, 45% abdominal mass, acute abdominal pain
Hemoperitoneum	Less than 1%	25%
Liver function tests	Nearly always normal	Nearly always normal
Malignant potential	Resection if operative risk negligible	Resection
II. Angiography		
Vascularity	Hypervascular with dense capillary blush	Hypervascular
Hematoma formation	Rare	Common
Necrosis	Rare	Common
Septation	Present in 50%	Absent
III. Liver scan		
Uptake	Normal or slightly decreased	None
IV. Pathology		
Capsule	No capsule	Partial to ample encapsulation
Location	Usually subscapular, 20% pedunculated	Usually subscapular, 7% pedunculated
Lesions	Often multiple	Usually solitary
Stellate scar	Present	Absent
Parenchyma	Nodular	Homogenous
Hemorrhage, necrosis	Rare	Common
Bile stasis	Absent	Present
Hepatocytes	Cytologically normal	Glycogen rich, vacuolated
Bile ductules	Present	Absent
Kupffer cells	Present	Reduced or absent
Vascularity	Large thick-walled vessels	Thin-walled sinusoids
Ultrastructure	Normal	Simplified

From Knowles DM II et al: *Medicine,* 57:223, 1978.

III-33   CLINICAL FEATURES OF HEPATOMA

I. General
   A. 80% to 90% of primary hepatic neoplasms are hepatic cell carcinomas (i.e., hepatoma); 10% are bile duct carcinomas (cholangiocarcinoma); approximately 70% of patients have underlying cirrhosis, most frequently postnecrotic or "mixed" type

II. Symptoms
   A. Common: weight loss, abdominal pain, anorexia, nausea, and emesis, which occur in 40% to 70% of patients
   B. Uncommon; fever, cough, hemoptysis

III. Physical Findings
   A. Common: hepatomegaly, ascites, jaundice, hepatic bruit, liver tenderness to palpation, edema
   B. Uncommon: splenomegaly, hepatic coma (except terminally), fever

IV. Atypical Presentations and Manifestations
   A. Acute cholecystitis syndrome
   B. Acute abdominal catastrophe (hemoperitoneum)
   C. Pulmonary embolism with or without infarction and malignant pleural effusion
   D. Budd-Chiari syndrome
   E. Erythrocytosis (~10% of patients)
   F. Hypercalcemia
   G. Hyperglycemia
   H. Hypercholesterolemia
   I. Fever of unknown origin

V. Diagnosis
   A. Clinical findings
      1. Unexplained deterioration in a cirrhotic*
      2. Hepatomegaly with a disproportionately ↑ serum alkaline phosphatase with no or little elevation in serum bilirubin*
      3. Hepatic bruit
      4. Elevated right hemidiaphragm

VI. Laboratory findings
   A. Abnormal liver scan/sonogram/CT scan
   B. Abnormal hepatic angiogram*
   C. Abnormal fibrinogen
   D. Positive liver biopsy (approximately 70% of cases)*
   E. Distant metastases

Continued

III-33   CLINICAL FEATURES OF HEPATOMA—*cont'd*

VII. Serologic tumor markers
  A. Alpha-fetoprotein (70% to 85% of cases)
  B. Hepatitis B markers in serum and liver (42% to 88% of cases)
  C. Vitamin B_{12} binding protein (7% of cases)
  D. Alpha$_1$-antitrypsin (5% of cases)
  E. Hepatitis C markers (40% to 70% of cases)
VIII. Course
  A. Average course is 4-8 months after onset of symptoms
  B. Generally poor responses to chemotherapy
  C. Gastrointestinal bleeding is common (35% to 50% of cases)
  D. Hepatic coma develops in 20% to 30% of cases

*Most important.

From Greenberger NJ: *Gastrointestinal disorders: A pathophysiological approach,* ed 4, Chicago, 1989, Year Book Medical Publishers, p. 391.

III-34   DIAGNOSIS OF WILSON'S DISEASE

  I. Abnormalities uniformly present
    *A. Kayser-Fleischer rings
    *B. Serum ceruloplasmin (< 20 mg/100 ml)
    *C. Urine copper excretion (> 100 µg/day)
    D. Liver copper content (> 250 µg/gm dry wt. of liver)
    E. Abnormal metabolism of ^{64}Cu
  II. Abnormalaties frequently present
    A. $\downarrow$ Serum uric acid and uricosuria
    B. Aminoaciduria
    C. Renal glycosuria
    D. Chronic active liver disease, cirrhosis
    E. Splenomegaly
    F. Thrombocytopenia
    G. Hemolytic anemia
  III. Central nervous system abnormalities

*These three items are used to screen for Wilson's disease.

From Greenberger NJ: *Gastrointestinal disorders: A pathophysiological approach,* ed 4, Chicago, 1989, Year Book Medical Publishers, p. 390.

III-35   PRINCIPAL ALTERATIONS OF HEPATIC MORPHOLOGY PRODUCED BY SOME COMMONLY USED DRUGS AND CHEMICALS

Principal morphologic change	Class of agent	Example
Cholestasis	Anabolic steroid	Methyl testosterone*
	Antithyroid	Methimazole
	Chemotherapeutic	Erythromycin estolate
	Oral contraceptive	Norethynodrel with mestranol
	Oral hypoglycemic	Chlorpropamide
	Tranquilizer	Chlorpromazine*
Fatty liver	Chemotherapeutic	Tetracycline
	Anticonvulsant	Valproic acid (sodium valproate)
Hepatitis	Anesthetic	Halothane†
	Anticonvulsant	Phenytoin
	Antihypertensive	Methyldopa†
	Chemotherapeutic	Isoniazid†
	Diuretic	Chlorothiazide
	Laxative	Oxyphenisatin†
Toxic (necrosis)	Hydrocarbon	Carbon tetrachloride
	Metal	Yellow phosphorus
	Mushroom	*Amanita phalloides*
	Analgesic	Acetaminophen
Granulomas	Anti-inflammatory	Phenylbutazone
	Chemotherapeutic	Sulfonamides
	Xanthine inhibitor	Allupurinol

*Rarely associated with primary biliary cirrhosis-like lesion.
†Occasionally associated with chronic active hepatitis or bridging hepatic necrosis and cirrhosis.
From Dienstag FL, Wands JR. In Braunwald E et al (eds): *Harrison's principles of internal medicine,* ed 11. New York, 1987, McGraw-Hill, p. 1336.

III-36   CAUSES OF PANCREATIC EXOCRINE INSUFFICIENCY

    I. Alcohol, chronic alcoholism
    II. Cystic fibrosis
    III. Severe protein calorie malnutrition with hypoalbuminemia
    IV. Pancreatic and duodenal neoplasms
    V. Pancreatic resection
    VI. Gastric surgery
        A. Subtotal gastrectomy with Billroth II anastomosis
        B. Subtotal gastrectomy with Billroth I anastomosis
        C. Truncal vagotomy with pyloroplasty
    VII. Gastrinoma (Zollinger-Ellison syndrome)
    VIII. Hereditary pancreatitis
    IX. Traumatic pancreatitis
    X. Hemochromatosis
    XI. Shwachman's syndrome (pancreatic insufficiency and bone marrow dysfunction)
    XII. Trypsinogen deficiency
    XIII. Enterokinase deficiency
    XIV. Radiation-induced chronic pancreatitis
    XV. Alpha$_1$-antitrypsin deficiency
    XVI. Idiopathic pancreatitis

From Greenberger NJ, Isselbacher KJ, Toskes PP. In *Harrison's principles of internal medicine,* ed 13. New York, 1994, McGraw-Hill, p. 1527.

III-37 CAUSES OF ACUTE PANCREATITIS

I. Alcohol ingestion (acute and chronic alcoholism)
II. Biliary tract disease (gallstones)
III. Postoperative (abdominal, nonabdominal)
IV. Postendoscopic retrograde cholangiopancraetography (ERCP)
V. Trauma (especially blunt abdominal trauma)
VI. Metabolic
   A. Hypertriglyceridemia
   B. Hyperparathyroidism
   C. Acute fatty liver of pregnancy
VII. Hereditary pancreatitis
VIII. Infections
   A. Mumps
   B. Viral hepatitis
   C. Mycoplasma
   D. Other viral infections (coxsackie and ECHO virus)
IX. Connective tissue disorders with vasculitis
   A. Systemic lupus erythematosus
   B. Necrotizing angiitis
   C. Thrombotic thrombocytopenic purpura
   D. Henoch-Schönlein purpura
X. Drug associated
   A. Definite association
      1. Azathioprine, 6-MP
      2. Sulfonamides
      3. Thiazide diuretics
      4. Furosemide
      5. Estrogens (oral contraceptives)
      6. Tetracycline
      7. Valproic acid
      8. DDI
      9. Pentamidine
      10. ACE inhibitors
   B. Probable association
      1. Chlorthalidone
      2. Ethacrynic acid
      3. Procainamide
      4. L-asparaginase
      5. Erythromycin
      6. Methyldopa
      7. Metronidazole
      8. NSAID's
   C. Equivocal association
      1. Corticosteroids
XI. Obstruction of the ampulla of Vater
   A. Regional enteritis
   B. Duodenal diverticulum
XII. Penetrating duodenal ulcer
XIII. Pancreas divisum

Continued

XIV. Recurrent bouts of acute pancreatitis without obvious cause
- A. Consider
  1. Occult disease of the gallbladder, biliary tree, pancreas, pancreatic ducts
  2. Drugs
  3. Hypertriglyceridemia
  4. Pancreas divisum
  5. Hereditary pancreatitis
  6. Pancreatic cancer
  7. Sphincter of Oddi dysfunction

From Greenberger NJ, Toskes P, Isselbacher KJ. Diseases of the pancreas. In *Harrison's principles of internal medicine,* ed 13, New York, 1994, McGraw-Hill, p. 1521.

III-38 **FACTORS ADVERSELY INFLUENCING SURVIVAL IN ACUTE PANCREATITIS***

I. Risk factors identifiable upon admission to hospital
- A. Increasing age
- B. Hypotension
- C. Tachycardia
- D. Abnormal physical examination of the lungs
- E. Abdominal mass
- F. Fever
- G. Leukocytosis
- H. Hyperglycemia
- I. First attack of pancreatitis
- J. Obesity (increased body mass index)

II. Risk factors identifiable during initial 48 hr of hospitalization
- A. Fall in hematocrit >10% with hydration and/or hematocrit <30%
- B. Necessity for massive fluid and colloid replacement
- C. Hypocalcemia
- D. Hypoxemia with or without adult respiratory distress syndrome
- E. Hypoalbuminemia
- F. Azotemia

III. Major risk factors†
- A. Hypotension
- B. Need for massive fluid and colloid replacement
- C. Respiratory failure
- D. Hypocalcemia
- E. Hemorrhagic peritoneal fluid

IV. Apache score >13

V. Multiorgan failure
- A. Respiratory (pO_2 <60)
- B. Renal (azotemia)
- C. Metabolic (hypocalcemia)
- D. Cardiovascular
- E. Central nervous system (obtundation)

*Increased mortality can be expected if 3 or more risk factors in Groups I and II are present.
†If 3 or more major risk factors from Group III are present, mortality rates can exceed 30%.

III-39   COMPLICATIONS OF ACUTE PANCREATITIS

I. Local
  A. Pancreatic phlegmon
  B. Pancreatic pseudocyst
    1. Pain
    2. Rupture with/without hemorrhage
    3. Hemorrhage
    4. Infection
  C. Pancreatic ascites
    1. Disruption of main pancreatic duct
    2. Leaking pseudocyst
  D. Pancreatic abscess
  E. Involvement of contiguous organs by necrotizing pancreatitis
    1. Massive intraperitoneal hemorrhage
    2. Thrombosis of blood vessels
    3. Bowel infarction
  F. Obstructive jaundice
II. Systemic
  A. Pulmonary
    1. Atelectasis
    2. Pneumonitis
    3. Pleural effusion
    4. Mediastinal abscess
    5. Adult respiratory distress syndrome
  B. Cardiovascular
    1. Hypotension
      a. hypovolemia
      b. hypoalbuminemia
    2. Sudden death
    3. Nonspecific ST-T changes in electrocardiogram simulating mycoardial infarction
    4. Pericardial effusion
  C. Hematologic
    1. Disseminated intravascular coagulation (DIC)
  D. Gastrointestinal hemorrhage
    1. Peptic ulcer disease
    2. Erosive gastritis
    3. Hemorrhagic pancreatic necrosis with erosion into major blood vessels
    4. Portal vein thrombosis; variceal hemorrhage
  E. Renal
    1. Oliguria } usually due to hypovolemia
    2. Azotemia
    3. Renal artery and/or renal vein thrombosis

Continued

III-39   COMPLICATIONS OF ACUTE PANCREATITIS—
   cont'd
   F. Metabolic
      1. Hyperglycemia
      2. Hypertriglyceridemia
      3. Hypocalcemia
   G. Central nervous system
      1. Psychosis
      2. Fat emboli
      3. Encephalopathy
   H. Fat necrosis
      1. Subcutaneous tissues/erythematous nodules
      2. Bone
      3. Other organs (mediastinum, pleura, nervous system)
   I. Miscellaneous
      1. Sudden blindness (Purtscher's retinopathy)

From Greenberger MJ, Toskes PP, Isselbacher KJ. In *Harrison's principles of internal medicine,* ed 13, New York, 1994, McGraw-Hill, p. 1524.

III-40   COMPLICATIONS OF CHRONIC PANCREATITIS
   I. Exocrine pancreatic insufficiency, steatorrhea, creatorrhea
   II. Vitamin B_{12} malabsorption
   III. Diabetes mellitus (difficult to exclude genetic diabetes)
   IV. Recurrent bouts of acute pancreatitis
   V. Pleural effusion (usually left-sided)
   VI. Pericardial effusion (rare)
   VII. Pancreatic ascites
      A. Disruption of pancreatic duct
      B. Leaking pseudocyst
   VIII. Altered mental status (psychosis, etc.)
   IX. Ischemic necrosis of bone and intramedullary calcification
   X. Common bile duct stenosis, obstructive jaundice, biliary cirrhosis
   XI. Addiction to narcotics and analgesics
   XII. ? Increased incidence of pancreatic carcinoma (no firm evidence for this)
   XIII. Non-diabetic retinopathy

III-41 DIAGNOSIS OF EXOCRINE PANCREATIC INSUFFICIENCY (EPI)

I. Identify etiology of EPI
II. Steatorrhea* with/without creatorrhea; $\uparrow$ stool N_2
III. Pancreatic calcification*
IV. Diabetes mellitus*
V. Test of pancreatic exocrine function†
    A. Secretin with/without CCK-PZ $\rightarrow$ $\downarrow$ volume [HCO_3], $\downarrow$ enzyme output
    B. Tripeptide test (Bentiromide) $\rightarrow$ $\downarrow$ urine excretion of Para-aminobenzoic acid (PABA)
    C. Other indirect pancreatic function tests
    D. $\downarrow$ serum trypsinogen, $\downarrow$ serum pancreatic isoamylase
VI. $\downarrow$ Absorption of vitamin B_{12}
VII. Normal tests of mucosal function (D-xylose, small bowel mucosal biopsy)
VIII. Response to pancreatic enzyme therapy
    A. Weight gain
    B. $\downarrow$ steatorrhea, creatorrhea

*Classical diagnostic triad.
†Frequently necessary as only ¼ patients with exocrine pancreatic insufficiency have the classical diagnostic triad.

III-42 POSTCHOLECYSTECTOMY SYNDROME

I. Definition: Persistence of abdominal pain after cholecystectomy
II. Causes
    A. Original diagnosis of cholecystitis/cholelithiasis as explanation for pain is incorrect
    B. Cholecystectomy not done or cholecystostomy performed
    C. Choledocholithiasis
        1. Stones missed at time of cholecystectomy
        2. Stones formed after cholecystectomy
    D. Common bile duct injury (stricture, etc.)
    E. Sclerosing cholangitis
    F. Bile duct carcinoma
    G. Chronic pancreatitis
    H. Sphincter of Oddi dysfunction
    I. Stenosis of papilla of Vater
    J. Anterior abdominal wall pain
        1. Scar tissue, traumatic neuroma, etc.

III-43   CRITERIA FOR ASSESSING SEVERITY OF MALNUTRITION

I. Anthropometric measurements
   A. Actual weight; ideal weight ($\downarrow$ <70% with severe malnutrition)
   B. Triceps skin fold thickness (reflects fat stores, severe depletion < 60%)
      1. Males—12.5 mm
      2. Females—16.5 mm
   C. Midarm muscle circumference (reflects protein stores, severe depletion < 60%)
      1. Males—25.3 cm
      2. Females—23.2 cm
II. Laboratory measurements
   A. Urinary creatinine (mg/24 hr): height (cm)
      1. Males—normal > 10.5
      2. Females—>5.8
   B. Serum albumin < 3.0 gm/dl
   C. Serum transferrin < 150 μg/dl
   D. Absolute lymphocyte count < 800/ml

III-44   DIFFERENTIAL DIAGNOSIS OF HYPOALBUMINEMIA

I. Chronic renal disease with nephrotic syndrome
II. Chronic parenchymal liver disease
III. Malabsorption
IV. Malnutrition
V. Protein-losing enteropathy
VI. Burns
VII. Eczematoid dermatitis (severe)
VIII. Analbuminemia (failure to synthesize albumin)

III-45   GRANULOMATOUS LIVER DISEASE

I. Infections
   A. Viral (cytomegalovirus, Epstein-Barr virus)
   B. Bacterial (Brucella, Q fever, Mycobacterium)
   C. Fungal (histoplasmosis, coccidiomycosis, cryptococcosis, candidiasis, aspergillosis)
   D. Parasites (ascariasis, schistosomiasis, amebiasis)
   E. Spirochetes (syphilis)
II. Drug induced
   A. Sulfonamides
   B. Procainamide
   C. Phenytoin
   D. Allupurinol
   E. Phenylbutazone
   F. Isoniazid
   G. Methyldopa
   H. Quinidine
   I. Halothane
   J. Carbamezepine
III. Neoplasms
   A. Hodgkin's disease
   B. Non-Hodgkin's lymphoma
IV. Miscellaneous
   A. Sarcoidosis
   B. Primary biliary cirrhosis
   C. Regional enteritis
   D. Berylliosis

III-46 DELTA AGENT*

I. General considerations
- A. Delta agent is a unique RNA virus which requires hepatitis B virus for its expression
- B. Delta infection has been transmitted to chimpanzees previously infected with hepatitis B virus
- C. Delta antibody has been measured in patients and is a reliable marker of Delta infection

II. Clinical aspects
- A. Delta agent + HBV infection (co-infection) usually results in an illness not different from classical hepatitis B
- B. Occasionally, co-infection can result in fulminant hepatitis
- C. Incidence of (+) Delta markers 20-50% in fulminant hepatitis
- D. Delta infection can aggravate pre-existing HBV liver disease or cause new disease in asymptomatic HB_sAg carriers
- E. Yucpa Indians—18% fulminant hepatitis with Delta infection; high HB_sAg carriage rate
- F. High incidence of Delta agent (60-80%) in patients with chronic HBV liver disease
- G. What determines fulminant or chronic cause of Delta hepatitis?
  1. Active HBV infection with HB_eAg associated with severe acute illness
  2. Inactive HBV infection with HB_eAg associated with chronicity
- H. Chronic hepatitis in 137 hepatitis B carriers and intrahepatic Delta antigen
  1. Fatal outcome in 12.8% with F/U 2-6 years
  2. 31/75 patients (41%) developed manifest cirrhosis in 2-6 years F/U

*Conclusion: Chronic delta infection worsens the histologic lesion and accelerates the course of liver disease.

From Greenberger NJ: *Gastrointestinal disorders: A pathophysiological approach,* ed 4, Chicago, 1989, Year Book Medical Publishers, p. 321.

III-47 PRIMARY SCLEROSING CHOLANGITIS
I. Definition:
   A. Obliterative inflammatory fibrosis of the extrahepatic bile ducts with or without intrahepatic duct involvement
II. Histologic features:
   A. ↓ Number of bile ducts
   B. Ductular proliferation
   C. Portal inflammation
   D. Substantial copper deposition
   E. Piecemeal necrosis
   F. Cirrhosis
III. Diseases associated with PSC
   A. Idiopathic ulcerative colitis (UC) (50% to 75%)
   B. Granulomatous colitis/ileocolitis (< 5%)
   C. Thyroiditis (< 5%)
   D. Pancreatitis (< 5%)
   E. Sicca syndrome (< 5%)
   F. Hypothyroidism (< 5%)
IV. Clinical features
   A. 70% are males
   B. Presenting features
      1. Jaundice
      2. Pruritis
      3. Abdominal pain
      4. Hepatosplenomegaly
      5. Abnormal liver tests
   C. May precede or follow IUC
   D. Mean survival ~ 5 years
   E. Death usually due to liver failure
   F. Copper overload ≃ PBC
   G. Screen for PSC in IUC patients with ↑ Alk. Phos.

PSC, primary sclerosing cholangitis; *PBC,* primary biliary cirrhosis; *IUC,* idiopathic ulcerative colitis.

From Greenberger NJ: *Gastrointestinal disorders: A pathophysiological approach,* ed 4, Chicago, 1989, Year Book Medical Publishers, p. 418.

III-48   PREDISPOSING FACTORS FOR CHOLESTEROL AND PIGMENT GALLSTONE FORMATION

I. Cholesterol and mixed stones
- A. Demography
  1. Northern Europe and North and South America greater than Orient; probably familial, hereditary aspects
- B. Obesity
  1. Normal bile acid secretion but ↑ biliary secretion of cholesterol
- C. Weight loss
  1. ↑ biliary cholesterol secretion while ↓ enteropathic secretion of bile salt
- D. Female sex hormones
  1. Estrogens stimulate ↑ liver uptake of dietary cholesterol, and ↑ biliary cholesterol.
  2. Oral contraceptives ↓ bile acid pool size and bile salt secretions
- E. Ileal disease or resection
  1. Malabsorption of bile acids leads to ↓ bile acid pool and ↓ biliary secretion of bile salts
- F. Increasing age
  1. ↑ biliary secretion of cholesterol, ↓ size of bile acid pool, ↓ biliary secretion of bile salts
- G. Gallbladder hypomotility leading to stasis and formation sludge
  1. Prolonged parenteral nutrition
  2. Fasting
  3. Pregnancy
  4. Drugs such as octreotide
- H. Clofibrate therapy
  1. ↑ biliary secretion of cholesterol

II. Pigment stones
- A. Demographic/genetic factors: orient, rural setting
- B. Chronic hemolysis
- C. Alcoholic cirrhosis
- D. Chronic biliary tract infection, parasite infestation
- E. Increasing age

III-49 CAUSES OF FULMINANT HEPATIC FAILURE

I. Infectious
   A. Common causes
      1. Viral hepatitis A, B, D, E
      2. Non-A, non-B (?C) hepatitis
   B. Rare causes
      1. Cytomegalovirus
      2. Epstein-Barr virus
      3. Herpes simplex virus
      4. Paramyxovirus (syncytial giant cell hepatitis)
II. Metabolic
   A. Acute fatty liver of pregnancy
   B. Reye's syndrome
III. Drugs/chemical exposure
   A. Carbon tetrachloride
   B. *Amanita phalloides* mushroom poisoning
   C. Acetaminophen overdose
   D. Tetracycline
   E. Halothane
   F. Sodium valproate
   G. Isoniazid
   H. Methyldopa
   I. Monoamine oxidase inhibitors
   J. Yellow phosphorus
   K. Nonsteroidal anti-inflammatory drugs
IV. Ischemic/hypoxic
   A. Hepatic arterial or venous occlusion
   B. Shock
   C. Hyperthermia
   D. Primary graft nonfunction post liver transplantation
V. Disorders presenting as fulminant hepatic failure with histological evidence of chronic liver disease
   A. Wilson's disease
   B. Massive malignant infiltration of the liver
   C. Liver failure postjejunoileal bypass
   D. Autoimmune chronic active hepatitis
   E. Chronic hepatitis B with reactivation or delta superinfection
   F. Erythropoietic protoporphyria

From Fingerote RJ, Bain VG: *Am J Gastro* 88:1000, 1993.

CHAPTER IV

Hematology-Oncology

IV-1   DIFFERENTIAL DIAGNOSIS OF NORMOCHROMIC-NORMOCYTIC ANEMIA

I. Primary bone marrow failure
   A. Aplastic anemia
   B. Myelophthisic anemia
      1. Leukemia and lymphoma
      2. Other neoplasms
      3. Myelofibrosis
      4. Granulomas
II. Secondary anemias
   A. Anemia of chronic inflammation
      1. Connective tissue disease
      2. Chronic infection
   B. Anemia of uremia
   C. Anemias associated with endocrinopathies
      1. Hypothyroidism
      2. Addison's disease
      3. Hypogonadism
      4. Panhypopituitarism
   D. Anemia associated with chronic liver disease
   E. Recent blood loss
   F. HIV infection
   G. Acute hemolysis

From Bunn HF. In Isselbacher KJ et al (eds): *Harrison's principles of internal medicine,* ed 10, New York, 1983, McGraw-Hill, p. 289.

IV-2 DIFFERENTIAL DIAGNOSIS OF MICROCYTIC-HYPOCHROMIC ANEMIA

I. Iron deficiency anemia
   A. Nutritional deficiency
   B. Chronic blood loss
   C. Gastric surgery and achlorhydria
   D. Improved absorption
   E. Increased requirements (e.g., pregnancy)
II. Sideroblastic anemia
   A. Hereditary or congenital
      1. X-linked
      2. Autosomal recessive
   B. Acquired sideroblastic anemia
      1. Idiopathic refractory sideroblastic anemia
      2. Secondary to underlying disease
         a. Neoplasms
         b. Inflammatory
         c. Hematologic
         d. Metabolic
      3. Associated with drugs or toxins
         a. Ethanol
         b. Lead
         c. Antituberculosis agents
         d. Chloramphenicol
         e. Alkylating agents
III. Thalassemia
IV. Chronic disease

From Lee GR, Wintrobe MM, Bunn FH. In Isselbacher KJ et al (eds): *Harrison's principles of internal medicine,* ed 9, New York, 1980, McGraw-Hill, pp. 1515-1517.

IV-3 DIFFERENTIAL DIAGNOSIS OF MACROCYTIC ANEMIAS

I. Vitamin B_{12} deficiency
   A. Inadequate intake (rare)
   B. Malabsorption
      1. Low intrinsic factor
         a. Pernicious anemia
         b. Postgastrectomy
         c. Congenital absence of intrinsic factor
      2. Disorders of terminal ileum
         a. Surgical resection
         b. Sprue
         c. Inflammatory bowel disease
         d. Neoplasms
         e. Granulomatous disease
         f. Selective cobalamin malabsorption (rare)

Continued

IV-3   DIFFERENTIAL DIAGNOSIS OF MACROCYTIC ANEMIAS—*cont'd*

3. Competition for vitamin B_{12}
   a. Fish tapeworm
   b. Bacteria: blind loop syndrome
4. Drugs
   a. *p*-Aminosalicylic acid
   b. Colchicine
   c. Neomycin

C. Transcobalamin II deficiency

II. Folate deficiency
   A. Inadequate intake
   B. Malabsorption
      1. Sprue
      2. Drugs (phenytoin, barbiturates)
   C. Increased requirements
      1. Pregnancy
      2. Infancy
      3. Malignancy
      4. Chronic hemolytic anemia
      5. Chronic exfoliative dermatitis
      6. Hemodialysis
   D. Impaired metabolism
      1. Drugs that inhibit dihydrofolate reductase (methotrexate, pentamidine, triamterene)
      2. Alcohol
      3. Enzyme deficiencies

III. Myelodysplastic syndromes

IV. Miscellaneous
   A. Chemotherapeutic agents which interfere with DNA metabolism
      1. 6-Mercaptopurine
      2. Azathioprine
      3. 5-Fluorouracil
      4. Cytosine arabinoside
      5. Procarbazine
      6. Hydroxyurea
      7. Acyclovir
      8. Zidovudine
   B. Spherocytosis
   C. Hypothyroidism
   D. Liver disease
   E. Reticulocytosis
   F. Hereditary orotic aciduria and other rare metabolic disorders
   G. DiGuglielmo's syndrome (acute erythroleukemia)

From Babior BM, Bunn HF. In Isselbacher KJ et al (eds): *Harrison's principles of internal medicine*, ed 13, New York, 1994, McGraw-Hill, p. 1726.

IV-4 DIFFERENTIAL DIAGNOSIS OF HEMOLYTIC ANEMIAS

I. Inherited disorders
- A. Defects in the erythrocyte membrane
  1. Hereditary spherocytosis
  2. Hereditary elliptocytosis
  3. Abetalipoproteinemia
  4. Hereditary stomatocytosis
  5. LCAT deficiency
- B. Deficiency of erythrocyte glycolytic enzymes
  1. Pyruvate kinase
  2. Hexokinase
  3. Aldolase
- C. Abnormalities of erythrocyte nucleotide metabolism
  1. Pyrimidine 5'nucleotidase deficiency
  2. Adenosine deaminase excess
  3. Adenosine triphosphatase deficiency
  4. Adenylate kinase deficiency
- D. Deficiencies of enzymes involved in the pentose phosphate pathway and in glutathione metabolism
  1. G-6PD
  2. Glutamyl-cysteine synthetase
  3. Glutathione synthetase
  4. Glutathione reductase
- E. Defects in globin structure and synthesis
  1. Sickle cell anemia
  2. Thalassemia major
  3. Hemoglobin H disease

II. Acquired disorders
- A. Immunohemolytic anemias
  1. Secondary to transfusion of incompatible blood
  2. Hemolytic disease of the newborn
  3. Due to warm reactive antibodies
     a. Idiopathic
     b. "Secondary"
        (1) Virus and mycoplasma infection
        (2) Lymphosarcoma and CLL
        (3) Other malignancies
        (4) Immune-deficiency states
        (5) SLE and other "autoimmune" disorders
        (6) Drug induced
  4. Due to cold reactive antibodies
     a. Cold hemagglutinin disease
     b. Paroxysmal cold hemoglobinuria

Continued

IV-4   DIFFERENTIAL DIAGNOSIS OF HEMOLYTIC ANEMIAS—*cont'd*

B. Traumatic and microangiopathic hemolytic anemias
   1. Prosthetic valves and other cardiac abnormalities
   2. Hemolytic-uremic syndrome
   3. Thrombotic thrombocytopenic purpura
   4. Disseminated intravascular coagulation
   5. Graft rejection
   6. Immune complex disease
C. Infectious agents
   1. Protozoan
      a. Malaria
      b. Toxoplasmosis
      c. Leishmaniasis
      d. Trypanosomiasis
   2. Bacterial
      a. Bartonellosis
      b. Clostridial infections
      c. Typhoid fever
      d. Cholera
D. Chemicals, drugs, and venoms
   1. Oxidant drugs and chemicals
      a. Naphthalene
      b. Nitrofurantoin
      c. Sulfonamides
   2. Non-oxidant chemicals
      a. Arsine
      b. Copper
      c. Water
   3. Associated with hemodialysis and uremia
   4. Venoms
E. Physical agents
   1. Thermal injury
F. Hypophosphatemia
G. "Spur cell" anemia in liver disease
H. Paroxysmal nocturnal hemoglobinuria
I. Vitamin E deficiency in newborns

From Wintrobe et al. In *Clinical hematology,* vol I, ed 9, Philadelphia, 1993, Lea & Febiger, p. 947.

IV-5   DIFFERENTIAL DIAGNOSIS OF PANCYTOPENIA

I.   Aplastic anemia

II.   Pancytopenia with normal or increased bone marrow cellularity
   A.   Myelodysplastic syndromes
   B.   Hypersplenism
   C.   Vitamin B_{12} or folate deficiency

III.   Bone marrow replacement
   A.   Hematologic malignancies
   B.   Nonhematologic metastatic tumor
   C.   Storage-cell disorders
   D.   Osteopetrosis
   E.   Myelofibrosis

IV.   Paroxysmal nocturnal hemoglobinuria

V.   Infections
   A.   HIV
   B.   Tuberculosis
   C.   Atypical mycobacterium
   D.   Fungal
   E.   Cytomegalovirus

From Rappeport JM, Bunn HF. In Isselbacher KJ et al (eds): *Harrison's principles of internal medicine,* ed 13, New York, 1994, McGraw-Hill, p. 1754.

IV-6   DIFFERENTIAL DIAGNOSIS OF APLASTIC ANEMIA

I. Idiopathic
II. Constitutional (Fanconi's anemia)
III. Chemical and physical agents
    A. Dose-related
        1. Chloramphenicol
        2. Benzene
        3. Ionizing irradiation
        4. Alkylating agents
        5. Antimetabolites (folic acid antagonists, purine and pyrimidine analogues)
        6. Mitotic inhibitors
        7. Anthracyclines
        8. Inorganic arsenicals
    B. Idiosyncratic
        1. Acetazolamide
        2. Arsenicals
        3. Barbiturates
        4. Chloramphenicol
        5. Gold
        6. Insecticides
        7. Phenothiazines
        8. Phenylbutazone
        9. Pyrimethamine
        10. Solvents
        11. Sulfa drugs
        12. Thiouracils
IV. Viral Infections
    A. Hepatitis (especially, HCV)
    B. Epstein-Barr
    C. Parvovirus
    D. HIV
    E. Cytomegalovirus
V. Immunologically mediated aplasia
VI. Pregnancy
VII. Paroxysmal nocturnal hemoglobinuria
VIII. Miscellaneous: SLE, pancreatitis, miliary tuberculosis, Simmonds' disease, viral infections

From Rappeport JM, Bunn HF. In Isselbacher KJ et al (eds): *Harrison's principles of internal medicine,* ed 13, New York, 1994, McGraw-Hill, p.1754.

IV-7 DIFFERENTIAL DIAGNOSIS OF NEUTROPENIA

I. Decreased production
  A. Hematologic diseases
    1. Aplastic anemia
    2. Cyclic neutropenia
    3. Leukemia
    4. Chediak-Hiyashi syndrome
    5. Myelodysplastic syndromes
    6. Chronic idiopathic neutropenia
  B. Drug-induced condition
    1. Agranulocytosis
    2. Myelotoxic drugs
  C. Malignancies with marrow invasion
  D. Nutritional deficiencies
    1. Vitamin B_{12}
    2. Folate
    3. Copper
  E. Infections
    1. Tuberculosis
    2. Typhoid
    3. Mononucleosis
    4. Malaria
    5. Brucellosis
    6. Tularemia
    7. Measles
    8. Viral hepatitis
    9. Histoplasmosis
    10. HIV
II. Peripheral destruction
  A. Autoimmune disorders
    1. Felty's syndrome
    2. SLE
  B. Splenic trapping
  C. Antineutrophil antibodies
III. Peripheral margination
  A. Overwhelming bacterial infection
  B. Hemodialysis
  C. Cardiopulmonary bypass

From Gallin JI. In Isselbacher KJ et al (eds): *Harrison's principles of internal medicine,*
ed 13, New York, 1994, McGraw-Hill, p. 332.

IV-8 DIFFERENTIAL DIAGNOSIS OF NEUTROPHILIA

I. Physiologic
   A. Exercise
   B. Epinephrine
   C. Pain, emotion, or stress
II. Infections
   A. Bacterial
   B. Fungal
   C. Viral (less common)
III. Inflammation
   A. Burns
   B. Tissue necrosis
      1. Myocardial infarction
      2. Pulmonary infarction
   C. Connective tissue disease
   D. Hypersensitivity states
IV. Metabolic disorders
   A. Diabetic ketoacidosis
   B. Acute renal failure
   C. Eclampsia
   D. Poisoning
V. Myeloproliferative diseases
VI. Miscellaneous
   A. Metastatic carcinoma
   B. Acute hemorrhage or hemolysis
   C. Glucocorticosteroids
   D. Lithium therapy
   E. Idiopathic
VII. Leukocyte adhesion protein deficiency

From Gallin JI. In Isselbacher KJ (eds): *Harrison's principles of internal medicine*, ed 13, New York, McGraw-Hill, 1994, p. 332.

IV-9 DIFFERENTIAL DIAGNOSIS OF EOSINOPHILIA

   I. Allergic disorders
      A. Hay fever
      B. Asthma
      C. Urticaria
  II. Drug reactions
      A. Iodine
      B. Aspirin
      C. Cephalosporins
      D. Sulfonamides
 III. Dermatologic disorders including:
      A. Pemphigus
      B. Dermatitis herpetiformis
 IV. Parasitic infections
      A. Trichinosis
      B. Echinococcus
      C. Strongyloides
   V. Pulmonary infiltrate with eosinophilia
  VI. Malignancy
      A. Hodgkin's disease
      B. Chronic myelogenous leukemia
      C. Mycosis fungoides
      D. Carcinoma of lung, stomach, pancreas, ovary, or uterus
 VII. Connective tissue disease
      A. Rheumatoid arthritis
      B. Dermatomyositis
      C. Periarteritis nodosa
      D. Vasculitis syndrome (leukocytoclastic, hypersensitivity)
VIII. Hypereosinophilic syndromes
      A. Loeffler's endocarditis
      B. Eosinophilic leukemia
  IX. Chronic granulomatosis disease (sarcoidosis)
   X. Miscellaneous
      A. Adrenal insufficiency
  XI. Idiopathic

From Gallin J I. In Isselbacher KJ et al (eds): *Harrison's principles of internal medicine,*
ed 13, New York, 1994, McGraw-Hill, p. 336.

IV-10   DIFFERENTIAL DIAGNOSIS OF BASOPHILIA

I. Hematologic disorders
   A. Hodgkin's disease
   B. Myeloproliferative diseases
      1. Chronic myelogenous leukemia
      2. Polycythemia vera
   C. Carcinoma
   D. Myelofibrosis
   E. Basophilic leukemia
II. Chronic inflammatory conditions
   A. Ulcerative colitis
   B. Chronic sinusitis
   C. Occasionally with nephrosis
III. Myxedema
IV. Infections
   A. Influenza
   B. Varicella
   C. Tuberculosis
V. Miscellaneous
   A. Mastocytosis
   B. Estrogen administration
   C. Drug hypersensitivity
   D. Radiation exposure

From Wintrobe MM et al (eds). In *Clinical hematology,* vol I, ed 8, Philadelphia, 1981, Lea & Febiger, pp.1300-1301.

IV-11   DISORDERS ASSOCIATED WITH MONOCYTOSIS

I. Hematologic disorders
- A. Hemopoietic stem cell disorders
  1. Preleukemia
  2. Acute myelogenous leukemia
  3. Chronic myelogenous leukemia
  4. Polycythemia vera
- B. Lymphocytic tumors
  1. Lymphoma
  2. Multiple myeloma
- C. Histiocytosis
- D. Hemolytic anemia
- E. ITP
- F. Chronic neutropenias
- G. Postsplenectomy

II. Inflammatory and immune disorders
- A. Collagen diseases
- B. Gastrointestinal disorders
  1. Ulcerative colitis
  2. Regional enteritis
  3. Sprue
  4. Alcoholic liver disease
- C. Sarcoidosis
- D. Infections

III. Miscellaneous conditions
- A. Hand-Schüller-Christian disease
- B. Glucocorticoids
- C. Parturition

From Lichtman R. In Williams WJ et al (eds): *Hematology*, ed 4, New York, 1990, McGraw-Hill, p.883.

IV-12   DIFFERENTIAL DIAGNOSIS OF ABNORMALITIES FOUND ON PERIPHERAL SMEAR

I. Basophilic stippling
- A. Lead poisoning
- B. Heavy metal poisoning
- C. Severe anemia

II. Howell-Jolly bodies
- A. Severe hemolytic anemia
- B. Pernicious anemia
- C. Leukemia
- D. Thalassemia
- E. Postsplenectomy

Continued

IV-12   DIFFERENTIAL DIAGNOSIS OF ABNORMALITIES FOUND ON PERIPHERAL SMEAR—*cont'd*

III. Pappenheimer bodies
    A. Thalassemia
    B. Lead poisoning
    C. Di Guglielmo's disease
IV. Heinz-Ehrlich bodies
    A. Glucose-6-PD-deficiency
    B. Drug-induced hemolytic anemias
  V. Spherocytes
    A. Autoimmune hemolytic anemia
    B. Congenital spherocytosis
 VI. Stomatocytes
    A. Acute alcohol (transient)
    B. Drugs (e.g., phenothiazines)
    C. Neoplastic, cardiovascular, hepatobiliary disease
    D. Hereditary
VII. Target cells
    A. Hemoglobin C disease or trait
    B. Thalassemia minor
    C. Iron deficiency anemia
    D. Liver disease
    E. Postsplenectomy
VIII. Ovalocytes
    A. Microcytic anemia
    B. Hereditary
    C. Megaloblastic anemias
 IX. Teardrop
    A. Spent polycythemia vera
    B. Myelofibrosis
    C. Thalassemia (especially homozygous β)
  X. Sickle cells
 XI. Acanthocytes
    A. Abetalipoproteinemia
    B. Postsplenectomy
    C. Fulminant liver disease
XII. Helmet
    A. DIC
    B. Severe valvular heart disease
    C. Prosthetic heart valves
    D. Microangiopathic hemolytic anemia
    E. Snake bite

From Wallach J. In *Interpretation of diagnostic tests,* ed 4, Boston, 1986, Little, Brown, pp. 120-122.

IV-13 DIFFERENTIAL DIAGNOSIS OF ERYTHROCYTOSIS

I. Erythrocytosis associated with a normal or reduced red cell mass (spurious)
 A. Acute or chronic hemoconcentration (relative)
 B. Spurious polycythemia (also called stress polycythemia or Gaisböck's syndrome)
II. Erythrocytosis associated with an elevated red cell mass (absolute polycythemia)
 A. Polycythemia vera
 B. Secondary polycythemia (increased erythropoietin production)
  1. Systemic hypoxia
   a. High altitude
   b. Cardiac disease with right to left shunt
   c. Chronic pulmonary disease
  2. Decreased blood oxygen carrying capacity, increase in carboxyhemoglobin or methemoglobin
  3. Impaired oxygen delivery, hemoglobin with increased oxygen affinity or congenital decreased red cell 2,3 diphosphoglycerate
  4. Local hypoxia–renal artery stenosis
  5. Autonomous erythropoietin production
   a. Tumors
    (1) Hypernephroma
    (2) Cerebella hemangioblastoma
    (3) Hepatoma
    (4) Uterine fibroids
    (5) Pheochromocytoma
    (6) Adrenal cortical adenoma
    (7) Ovarian carcinoma
   b. Renal disorders
    (1) Cysts
    (2) Hydronephrosis
    (3) Bartter's syndrome
    (4) Transplantation
  6. Familial polycythemia due to autonomous erythropoietin production

From Hoffman R et al (eds). In Stollerman GH (ed): *Advances in internal medicine,* vol 24, Chicago, 1979, Yearbook Medical Publishers, p.260.

IV-14 CRITERIA FOR THE DIAGNOSIS OF POLYCYTHEMIA VERA

I. Major criteria
   A. Increased red cell mass
   B. Arterial O_2 saturation $\geq 92\%$
   C. Splenomegaly
II. Minor criteria
   A. Thrombocytosis
   B. Leukocytosis
   C. Elevated serum B_{12}
   D. Increased leukocyte alkaline phosphatase
   E. Increased serum B_{12} (>900 pg/ml) or unbound B_{12} binding capacity (>2200 pg/ml)

Diagnosis of polycythemia vera is made if patient has all three major criteria *or* the first two major criteria and any two minor criteria.

III. Most common presenting symptoms of patients in the national polycythemia vera study

Symptoms	Percentage
Headache	49
Weakness	47
Pruritus	46
Dizziness	45
Sweating	33
Weight loss	31
Paresthesias	29
Joint symptoms	28
Epigastric distress	28

From Berlin NI: Diagnosis and classification of polycythemias, *Semin Hematol* 12:339, 1975.

IV-15 DIFFERENTIAL DIAGNOSIS OF THROMBOCYTOSIS

   I. Myeloproliferative disorders
     A. Primary thrombocythemia
     B. Polycythemia vera
     C. Chronic myelogenous leukemia
     D. Agnogenic myeloid metaplasia
   II. Chronic inflammatory disorders
     A. Rheumatoid arthritis
     B. Acute rheumatic fever
     C. Polyarteritis nodosa
     D. Wegener's granulomatosis
     E. Ulcerative colitis
     F. Regional enteritis
     G. Tuberculosis
     H. Hepatic cirrhosis
     I. Sarcoidosis
  III. Acute hemorrhage
  IV. Iron deficiency anemia
   V. Hemolytic anemia
  VI. Malignancy
 VII. Postsplenectomy
VIII. Response to drugs
     A. Vincristine
     B. Epinephrine
  IX. Response to exercise
   X. Osteoporosis

From Williams WJ. In Williams WJ et al (eds): *Hematology,* ed 4, New York, 1990, McGraw-Hill, p. 1403.

IV-16 MYELODYSPLASTIC SYNDROMES

   I. Refractory anemia
  II. Refractory anemia with ringed sideroblasts
 III. Refractory anemia with excess blasts
 IV. Refractory anemia with excess blasts in transformation
   V. Chronic myelomonocytic leukemia

IV-17 MYELOPROLIFERATIVE SYNDROMES

   I. Chronic myelogenous leukemia
  II. Polycythemia vera
 III. Myelofibrosis
 IV. Essential thrombocythemia

IV-18   STAGING OF CHRONIC LYMPHOCYTIC LEUKEMIA

I. Rai classification
   - 0   Lymphocytosis >15,000 mm^3; marrow 40% lymphocyte
   - 1   Lymphocytosis plus lymphadenopathy
   - 2   Lymphocytosis plus hepatomegaly or splenomegaly
   - 3   Lymphocytosis plus anemia
   - 4   Lymphocytosis plus thrombocytopenia

II. Median survival of Rai classes
   - 0   >150 months
   - 1   105 months
   - 2   71 months
   - 3   19 months
   - 4   19 months

III. International staging
   - A   Lymphocytosis alone with fewer than 3 lymph node groups enlarged
   - B   Lymphocytosis with 3 or more lymph node groups enlarged
   - C   Lymphocytosis with anemia (hgb <10g/dl) or thrombocytopenia (plt <100,000 mm^3)

From Mitus AJ, Rosenthal DS. In Holleb AI, Fink DJ, Murphy GP (eds): *Clinical oncology,* Atlanta, 1991, p. 425.

IV-19   CRITERIA FOR THE DIAGNOSIS OF MULTIPLE MYELOMA

I. Major criteria
   - A. Plasmacytoma
   - B. IgG paraprotein >3.5 gm%
        IgA paraprotein >2 gm%
        Light chain in urine >1 gm%
   - C. Bone marrow plasma cells >30%

II. Minor criteria
   - A. Bone marrow plasma cells 10% to 30%
   - B. IgG paraprotein <3.5 gm%
        IgA paraprotein <2 gm%
   - C. Lytic bone lesions
   - D. Hypogammaglobulinemia (IgA <100 µg/dl, IgM <50 µg/dl)

III. To make the diagnosis (one of the following)
   - A. IA + either IIB, IIC, or IID
   - B. IB + either IIA, IIC, or IID
   - C. IC
   - D. IIA + IIB + IIC or IIA + IIB + II D

IV-20 STAGING SYSTEM FOR MULTIPLE MYELOMA

Stage	Criteria	Measured myeloma cell mass (cells on $10^{12}/m^2$)

I	All of the following:
	Hemoglobin value >10 g/dl
	Serum calcium value >12 mg/dl
	On x-ray: normal bone structure
	  (scale 0) or solitary osseous myeloma
	Low M component level
	  IgG <5 g/dl
	  IgA <3 g/dl
	  Urine light chain M component
	    <4 g/24h
		<0.6 (low)

II	Fitting between stage I and stage III	0.6-1.2 (intermediate)

III	One or more of the following:
	Hemoglobin value <8.5 g/dl
	Serum calcium value >12 mg/dl
	Advanced lytic bone lesions (scale 3)
	High M component level
	  IgG >7 g/dl
	  IgA >5 g/dl
	  Urine light chain M component
	    >12 g/24h
		≥1.2 (high)

SUBCLASSIFICATION

A Relatively normal renal function (serum creatinine value <2 mg/dl)
B Abnormal renal function (serum creatinine value >2 mg/dl)

From Jandl J: In *Blood: Textbook of hematology,* Boston, 1987, Little, Brown.

IV-21   RENAL AND ELECTROLYTE DISORDERS IN MULTIPLE MYELOMA
I. "Myeloma kidney"
II. Renal tubular dysfunction
III. Acute renal failure
IV. Amyloidosis
V. Plasma cell invasion of the kidneys
VI. Hypercalcemia
VII. Hyperuricemia
VIII. Spurious hyponatremia
IX. Urinary tract infections
X. Proteinuria
XI. Absence of hypertension

IV-22   CRITERIA FOR THE DIAGNOSIS OF THROMBOTIC THROMBOCYTOPENIC PURPURA
I. Fever
II. Microangiopathic hemolytic anemia* (Coombs negative)
III. Thrombocytopenia
IV. Neurologic disorders
V. Renal dysfunction

*Schistocytes on peripheral blood smear.

IV-23 DIFFERENTIAL DIAGNOSIS OF SPLENOMEGALY

I. Infections
   A. Mononucleosis
   B. Bacterial septicemia
   C. Tuberculosis
   D. Malaria
   E. Viral hepatitis
   F. AIDS
   G. Congenital syphilis
   H. Splenic abscess
   I. Disseminated histoplasmosis
   J. Bacterial endocarditis
   K. Leishmaniasis
   L. Trypanosomiasis

II. Disordered immunoregulation
   A. Rheumatoid arthritis (Felty's syndrome)
   B. Systemic lupus erythematosus
   C. Immune hemolytic anemia
   D. Angioimmunoblastic lymphadenopathy
   E. Drug reactions with serum sickness
   F. Immune thrombocytopenia and neutropenia

III. Altered splenic blood flow
   A. Luennec's and postnecrotic cirrhosis
   B. Hepatic vein obstruction
   C. Portal vein obstruction
   D. Congestive heart failure
   E. Splenic artery aneurysm
   F. Splenic vein obstruction

IV. Abnormal erythrocytes
   A. Spherocytosis
   B. Sickle cell disease
   C. Thalassemia
   D. Ovalocytes

V. Infiltrative diseases
   A. Benign: amyloidosis, Gaucher's disease, Niemann-Pick disease, Hurler syndrome, extramedullary hematopoiesis, splenic cysts.
   B. Malignant: leukemias, lymphomas, myeloproliferative syndromes, angiosarcoma, metastatic tumors.

VI. Miscellaneous
   A. Thyrotoxicosis
   B. Iron deficiency anemia
   C. Sarcoidosis
   D. Berylliosis

From Haynes B. In Isselbacher KJ et al (eds): *Harrison's principles of internal medicine,* ed 13, New York, 1994, McGraw-Hill, p. 327.

IV-24 DIFFERENTIAL DIAGNOSIS OF LYMPHADENOPATHY

I. Infectious diseases
   A. Viral
      1. HIV
      2. Mononucleosis
      3. Cytomegalovirus
      4. Infectious hepatitis
   B. Bacterial
      1. Pyogenic streptococcal or staphylococcal
      2. Brucellosis
   C. Fungal
      1. Histoplasmosis
      2. Coccidioidomycosis
   D. Mycobacterial
   E. Parasitic
      1. Toxoplasmosis
      2. Malaria
   F. Spirochetal
   G. Chlamydial infections
      1. Lymphogranuloma venereum
II. Immunologic diseases
   A. Rheumatoid arthritis
   B. Systemic lupus erythematosus
   C. Dermatomyositis
   D. Serum sickness
   E. Drug reactions
   F. Angioimmunoblastic lymphadenopathy
   G. Primary biliary cirrhosis
III. Malignant diseases
   A. Hematologic
      1. Lymphoma
      2. Malignant histiocytosis
      3. Acute leukemia
      4. Myeloproliferative syndromes
      5. Chronic lymphocytic leukemia
   B. Metastatic tumors to lymph nodes
IV. Endocrine diseases: hyperthyroidism
V. Lipid storage diseases
   A. Gaucher's disease
   B. Niemann-Pick disease
VI. Miscellaneous
   A. Sinus histiocytosis
   B. Sarcoidosis
   C. Amyloidosis
   D. Lymphomatoid granulomatosis
   E. Mucocutaneous lymph node syndrome
   F. Giant (angiofollicular) lymph node hyperplasia
   G. Dermatopathic lymphadenitis

From Haynes B. In Isselbacher KJ et al (eds): *Harrison's principles of internal medicine,* ed 13, New York, 1994, McGraw-Hill, p. 324.

IV-25 DIFFERENTIAL DIAGNOSIS OF THROMBOCYTOPENIA

I. Decreased marrow production
   A. Marrow infiltration with tumor, fibrosis
   B. Marrow failure: aplastic and hypoplastic anemias
   C. ? HIV
II. Splenic sequestration
   A. Splenic hypertrophy: tumor, portal hypertension
III. Increased destruction
   A. Nonimmune
      1. Vascular prostheses, cardiac valves
      2. DIC
      3. Sepsis
      4. Vasculitis
      5. Thrombotic thrombocytopenia purpura
   B. Immune
      1. Autoantibodies to platelet antigens (e.g., ITP)
      2. Drug-associated antibodies
      3. Circulatory immune complexes: lupus, viral agents, bacterial sepsis
      4. HIV

From Handin R. In Isselbacher KJ et al (eds): *Harrison's principles of internal medicine,* ed 13, New York, 1994, McGraw-Hill, pp. 1798-1799.

IV-26 CAUSES OF CYANOSIS

I. Central cyanosis
   A. Decreased arterial oxygen saturation
      1. Decreased atmospheric pressure-high altitude
      2. Impaired pulmonary function
         a. Alveolar hypoventilation
         b. Pulmonary ventilation/perfusion mismatching
         c. Impaired oxygen diffusion
      3. Anatomic shunts
         a. Certain types of congenital heart disease
         b. Pulmonary arteriovenous fistulas
         c. Multiple small intrapulmonary shunts
      4. Hemoglobin with low affinity for oxygen
   B. Hemoglobin abnormalities
      1. Methemoglobinemia-hereditary, acquired
      2. Sulfhemoglobinemia-acquired
      3. Carboxyhemoglobinemia (not true cyanosis)
II. Peripheral cyanosis
   A. Reduced cardiac output
   B. Cold exposure
   C. Redistribution of blood flow from extremities
   D. Arterial obstruction
   E. Venous obstruction

From Braunwald E. In Isselbacher KJ et al (eds): *Harrison's principles of internal medicine,* ed 13, New York, 1994, McGraw-Hill, p. 182.

IV-27   PARANEOPLASTIC SYNDROMES

  I. Endocrine
    *A. Cushing's syndrome
    *B. Hypercalcemia
    *C. Gynecomastia
     D. Hypoglycemia
     E. Hypokalemia
    *F. SIADH
     G. Carcinoid syndrome
     H. Hyperthyroidism
     I. Hypocalcemia
 II. Skeletal
    *A. Digital clubbing
    *B. Hypertrophic pulmonary osteoarthropathy
     C. Hyperpigmentation
III. Skin
    *A. Dermatomyositis
    *B. Acanthosis nigricans
 IV. Neurology
    *A. Eaton-Lambert syndrome
    *B. Peripheral neuropathies
    *C. Subacute cerebellar degeneration
     D. Cortical degeneration
     E. Polymyositis
     F. Transverse myelitis
     G. Progressive multifocal leukoencephalopathy
    *H. Encephalomyelitis
  V. Vascular
    *A. Thrombophlebitis
    *B. Marantic endocarditis
    *C. TTP
 VI. Hematology
    *A. Anemia
     B. Dysproteinemia
    *C. DIC
     D. Eosinophilia
    *E. Leukocytosis
     F. Erythrocytosis
    *G. Thrombocytosis
     H. Thrombocytopenia
VII. Other
     A. Nephrotic syndrome
     B. Hypouricemia

*Associated with bronchogenic carcinoma.

IV-28   CAUSES OF HYPONATREMIA IN CANCER PATIENTS

I. Pseudohyponatremia (multiple myeloma, other paraproteinemias)
II. Adrenal insufficiency
III. Gastrointestinal losses with "pure water" replacement
IV. SIADH
    A. Tumor-related (usually small cell carcinoma of the lung)
    B. Drug-related (cyclophosphamide, vinca alkaloids, narcotic analgesics, phenothiazines, barbiturates, tricyclic antidepressants)
    C. Infection-related (pulmonary and central nervous system infections)
    D. Central nervous system (Space-occupying lesions, infections)

IV-29   FACTORS RELATED TO THE SURVIVAL OF PATIENTS WITH BREAST CANCER

I. Disease-free survival related to lymph node status*

Axillary nodes	Surviving disease free (%)	
	At 5 yr	*At 10 yr*
Negative	83	76
1-3 Nodes positive	50	35
≥4 Nodes positive	21	11

II. Recurrence risk with negative nodes†
  I. Low risk
    A. Ductal carcinoma in situ, pure tubular, papillary, or typical medullary types
    B. Tumor <1 cm
    C. Diploid tumor; low S-phase fraction
  II. High risk
    A. Aneuploid tumor
    B. High S-phase fractions
    C. High cathepsin D levels
    D. Absent estrogen receptors
    E. Tumor >3 cm

*From National Surgical Adjuvant Breast Project.
†From McGuire R, Clark G: *N Engl J Med* 326(26):1757, 1992.

IV-30   TNM NOMENCLATURE AND STAGES OF LUNG CANCERS

T x   Positive sputum with normal X-ray

T o   No primary tumor identified

T   Carcinoma in situ
  1   Intraparenchymal tumor 3.0 cm or less in diameter
  2   Tumor more than 3 cm in diameter and/or invading visceral pleural or a main bronchus
  3   Any size tumor which invades chest wall, diaphragm, or mediastinal pleura, parietal pericardium or within 2 cm of carina but not involving the carina
  4   Any size tumor involving heart, great vessels, esophagus, or carina, or presence of a malignant pleural effusion

N 0   No proven involvement of any lymph node
  1   Peribronchial or ipsilateral hilar node involvement
  2   Ipsilateral mediastinal or subcarinal nodes involved
  3   Contralateral mediastinal/hilar nodes, ipsilateral or contralateral scalene or supraclavicular nodes involved

M 0   No evidence of distant metastasis
  1   Distant metastasis, e.g., bone, brain, liver, etc.

Stage 0
$T_xN_0M_0$ Occult carcinoma

*Stage 1
$T_{1-2}N_0M_0$ No lymph node involvement

*Stage II
$T_{1-2}N_1M_0$ Intrapulmonary and/or hilar nodes involved

*Stage IIIa
$T_{3-2}N_2M_0$ >3 cm tumor with only peribronchial or ipsilateral hilar nodes in-
$T_3N_{0-2}M_0$ volved; any size tumor not involving mediastinum with only ipsilateral or subcarinal node involvement

Stage IIIb
$T_4N_{0-2}M_0$ Any size tumor involving mediastinum or with contralateral node
$T_{1-4}N_3M_0$ involvement

Stage IV
$T_{x-4}N_{0-3}M_1$ Distant metastasis

*Considered potentially resectable.

From Faber LP. In Holleb AI, Fink DJ, Murphy GP (eds): *Clinical oncology,* ed. 1, Atlanta, 1991, p. 201.

IV-31 FAB CLASSIFICATION OF ACUTE MYELOGENOUS LEUKEMIA

Subtype	Features	Prognosis
MO Acute myeloblastic with no maturation	No granules	Good
M1 Acute myeloblastic with minimal maturation	Few granules	Good
M2 Acute myeloblastic with maturation	t(8;21), chloromas	Good
M3 Acute promyelocytic	t(15;17) DIC	Good
M4 Acute myelomonocytic	*Inv 16 esosinophils	Good
M5a Acute monoblastic without differentiation	t(9;11), extra-medullary disease	Poor
M5b Acute monoblastic with differentiation	Older patients than those with M5a	Poor
M6 Acute erythroleukemia	Bone pain, older patient Aneuploidy	Poor
M7 Megakaryocytic	Down syndrome association	Poor

t, Chromosome translocation.
*Inversion chromosome 16.

IV-32 MOST FREQUENT TYPES OF NEOPLASMS IN MALIGNANT PLEURAL EFFUSIONS

   I. Breast
  II. Lung
 III. Lymphoma/leukemia
  IV. Ovary
   V. Unknown primary
  VI. GI tract
 VII. Mesothelioma
VIII. Uterus
  IX. Kidney
   X. Sarcoma

From Papac RJ. In Becker FF (ed): *Cancer: A comprehensive treatise*, vol 5, New York, 1977, Plenum Press, p.208.

IV-33   MOST FREQUENT MALIGNANCIES CAUSING PERITONEAL EFFUSIONS

I. Ovary
II. Stomach
III. Uterus
IV. Unknown primary
V. Breast
VI. Lymphoma
VII. Mesothelioma

From Papac RJ. In Becker FF (ed): *Cancer: A comprehensive treatise,* Plenum Press, New York, 1977, Vol. 5, p.212.

IV-34   MOST FREQUENT NEOPLASMS CAUSING MALIGNANT PERICARDIAL EFFUSION

I. Leukemia, lymphoma
II. Breast
III. Lung
IV. Skin (melanoma)

From Papac RJ. In Becker FF (ed): *Cancer: A comprehensive treatise,* vol 5, New York, 1977, Plenum Press, p.214.

IV-35   ETIOLOGIC FACTORS OF HYPERCALCEMIA OF MALIGNANCY

I. Humoral factors
  A. Parathyroid hormone (PTH): rare
  B. PTH-related peptide
  C. Transforming growth factors (TGFα, TGFβ, IL-1)
  D. Prostaglandins
  E. Tumor necrosis factors
  F. Platelet-derived growth factor
  G. Colony-stimulating factors
  H. 1,25 dihydroxyvitamin D (with certain lymphomas)
II. Other causes
  A. Direct bone resorption by tumor-rare
  B. Increased GI absorption of calcium-rare
  C. Increased renal reabsorption of calcium

From Warrell R, Bockman R. In *Cancer: Principles of oncology,* ed 3, 1989, p. 1988.

IV-36   CANCERS MOST LIKELY TO METASTASIZE TO BONE

I. Thyroid
II. Breast
III. Prostate
IV. Renal
V. Lung

IV-37 GENERAL RESPONSES OF VARIOUS MALIGNANCIES TO ANTINEOPLASTIC CHEMOTHERAPY

I. Chemotherapy potentially curative
  A. Acute lymphocytic leukemia of childhood
  B. Burkitt's lymphoma
  C. Gestational trophoblastic neoplasia
  D. Hodgkin's disease
  E. Non-Hodgkin's lymphomas (diffuse large cell, nodular lymphocytic, nodular mixed types)
  F. Testicular tumors
  G. Embryonal rhabdomyosarcoma of childhood
  H. Ewing's sarcoma
  I. Wilms' tumor
  J. Acute nonlymphocytic leukemia
  K. Ovarian carcinomas

II. Chemotherapy palliative
  A. Adrenal carcinoma
  B. Acute lymphocytic leukemia of adults
  C. Acute nonlymphocytic leukemia
  D. Breast carcinoma
  E. Chronic myelogenous leukemia
  G. Endometrial carcinoma
  H. Gastric carcinoma
  I. Glioblastoma (few percent)
  J. Islet cell tumors
  K. Medullary carcinoma of the thyroid
  L. Multiple myeloma
  M. Neuroblastoma
  N. Non-Hodgkin's lymphomas
  O. Osteosarcoma
  P. Ovarian carcinoma
  Q. Prostatic carcinoma
  R. Bronchogenic carcinomas
  S. Soft-tissue sarcomas
  T. Bladder carcinoma
  U. Head and neck carcinomas
  V. Colorectal carcinoma

III. Chemotherapy marginally or questionably beneficial
  A. Biliary tract carcinoma
  B. Brain tumors
  C. Carcinoid tumors
  D. Cervical carcinoma
  E. Hepatocellular carcinoma
  F. Malignant melanoma
  G. Pancreatic carcinoma
  H. Renal cell carcinoma
  I. Thyroid carcinoma

From Moosa A, Robson M, Schimpff J: *Comprehensive textbook of oncology,* ed 2, Baltimore, 1991, Williams & Wilkins, p. 528.

IV-38 LONG-TERM EFFECTS OF RADIATION

  I. Salivary gland: Xerostomia
  II. Esophagus: Ulcer, stricture
  III. Stomach: Achlorhydria, pyloric stenosis, ulceration
  IV. Small intestine: Ulcer, perforation, stricture, malabsorption
  V. Colon: Ulcer, perforation, stricture, fistula formation
  VI. Kidney: Nephritis
  VII. Bladder: Ulceration, contracture, dysuria, frequency
  VIII. Lung: Pneumonitis, fibrosis
  IX. Heart: Pericarditis, pancarditis
  X. Bone: Arrested growth in children
  XI. CNS: Atrophy
  XII. Spinal cord: Transverse myelitis

From Becker FF (ed): *Cancer: A comprehensive treatise,* vol 5, New York, 1977, Plenum Press, p.8.

IV-39 CLINICAL FEATURES OF GRAFT-VS.-HOST DISEASE

  I. Suggested clinical staging

Stage	Skin	Liver	Intestinal Tract
+	Maculopapular rash <25% body surface	Serum bilirubin 2-3 mg/dl	>500 ml stool volume/day
+ +	Maculopapular rash 25-50% body surface	Serum bilirubin 3-6 mg/dl	>1000 ml stool volume/day
+ + +	Generalized erythroderma	Serum bilirubin 6-15 mg/dl	>1500 ml stool volume/day
+ + + +	Generalized erythroderma; bullous formation; desquamation	Serum bilirubin >15 mg/dl	Severe abdominal pain; ileus

  II. Suggested overall clinical grading

Grade	Skin	Liver	GI tract	Survival
I	+ – + +	0	0	>50%
II	+ – + + +	+	+	
III	+ + – + + +	+ + – + + +	+ + – + + +	15%
IV	+ + – + + + +	+ + – + + + +	+ + – + + + +	15%

From Thomas ED: *New Engl J Med* 292:895, 1975.

IV-40   SUPERIOR VENA CAVA SYNDROME

   I. Neoplasm
       A. 90% lung carcinoma
       B. 10% lymphoma
  II. Mediastinitis
       A. Fibrosing (TB, histoplasmosis, syphilis, pyogenic)
       B. Idiopathic
       C. Methysergide
 III. Aortic aneurysm
  IV. Thrombophlebitis
   V. Constrictive pericarditis
  VI. Retrosternal thyroid
 VII. Central venous catheters

IV-41   CAUDA EQUINA SYNDROME

   I. Perineal, buttock, leg pain
  II. Sphincteric incontinence
 III. Loss of sensation in perineum, posterior thigh, lateral feet
  IV. ↓ DTRs
   V. Foot drop
  VI. Impotence

IV-42   SIGNS AND SYMPTOMS OF METASTATIC EPIDURAL COMPRESSION

   I. Pain—96%
  II. Weakness—76%
 III. Autonomic dysfunction—57%
  IV. Sensory disturbances—51%
   V. Ataxia—3%
  VI. Flexor spasms—2%

From Byrne T: *N Engl J Med* 327(6):614, 1992.

IV-43 COTSWOLD STAGING CLASSIFICATION OF HODGKIN'S DISEASE

Stage	
I	Single lymph node region or lymphoid structure involved
II	Two or more lymph node regions on the same side of the diaphragm involved (number of anatomic sites indicated by a subscript)
III	Lymph node regions on both sides of the diaphragm involved
III_1	With or without splenic, hilar, celiac, or portal node involvement
III_2	Para-aortic, iliac, and mesenteric nodes involved
IV	One or more extranodal sites involved (in addition to a site for which the designation "E" has been used)

Designation	
A	No symptoms
B	Fever (>38°C), night sweats, unexplained weight loss >10% within last 6 months
X	Bulky disease (widening of mediastinum by more than one-third or a nodal mass greater than 10 cm)
E	Involvement of a single extranodal site that is contiguous or proximal to the known nodal site

From Urbu W, Longo D: *N Engl J Med* 326(10):679, 1992.

IV-44 WORKING FORMULATION OF NON-HODGKIN'S LYMPHOMAS

	Rappeport terminology
LOW GRADE	
1. Malignant lymphoma	
Small lymphocytic	DWDL
Consistent with chronic lymphocytic leukemia	
2. Malignant lymphoma, follicular	
Predominantly small cleaved cell	NPDL
Diffuse areas	
Sclerosis	
3. Malignant lymphoma, follicular	
Mixed, small cleaved, and large cell	NML
Diffuse areas	
Sclerosis	
INTERMEDIATE GRADE	
4. Malignant lymphoma, follicular	
Predominantly large cell	NHL
Diffuse areas	
Sclerosis	
5. Malignant lymphoma, diffuse	
Small cleaved cell	DPDL
Sclerosis	
6. Malignant lymphoma, diffuse	
Mixed, small, and large cell	DML
Sclerosis	
Epitheloid-cell component	
7. Malignant lymphoma, diffuse	
Large cell	DHL
Cleaved cell	
Noncleaved cell	
Sclerosis	
HIGH GRADE	
8. Malignant lymphoma	
Large cell, immunoblastic	DHL
Plasmacytoid	
Clear cell	
Polymorphous	
Epithelioid-cell component	
9. Malignant lymphoma	
Lymphoblastic	Lymphoblastic
Convoluted cell	
Nonconvoluted cell	

Continued

10. Malignant lymphoma
    Small noncleaved cell   DUL
        Burkitt's
        Follicular areas
    Miscellaneous
        Composite
        Histiocytic
        Extramedullary plasmacytoma
        Unclassifiable
        Other

From Moose A, Robson M, Schimpff J: *Comprehensive textbook of oncology*, Baltimore, 1986, Williams & Wilkins, p.577.

DWDL, Diffuse, well-differentiated, lymphocyic; *NPDL,* nodular, poorly-diffeentiated, lymphocytic; *NML,* nodular, mixed lymphocytic-histiocytic; *NHL,* nodular histiocytic; *DPDL,* diffuse, poorly-differentiated, lymphocytic; *DML,* diffuse, mixed lymphocytic-histiocytic; *DHL,* diffuse histioytic; *DUL,* undifferentiated.

IV-45   PERFORMANCE STATUS (KARNOFSKY SCALE)

Criteria of performance status

Able to carry on normal activity; no special care needed	100 Normal; no complaints; no evidence of disease
	90 Able to carry on normal activity; minor signs of symptoms of disease
	80 Normal activity with some effort; some signs or symptoms of disease
Unable to work; able to live at home and care for most personal needs; a varying amount of assistance is needed	70 Cares for self; unable to carry on normal activity or to do active work
	60 Requires occasional care for most needs
	50 Requires considerable assistance and frequent medical care
Unable to care for self; requires equivalent of institutional or hospital care; disease may be progressing rapidly	40 Disabled; requires special care and assistance
	30 Severely disabled; hospitalization indicated, although death not imminent
	20 Very sick; hospitalization; active supportive treatment is necessary
	10 Moribund, fatal processes progressing rapidly
	0 Dead

From Moose A, Robson M, Schimpff J: *Comprehensive textbook of oncology*, Baltimore, 1986, Williams & Wilkins, p.67.

IV-46   MULTIPLE ENDOCRINE NEOPLASIA SYNDROME

I. Multiple endocrine neoplasia type I (MEN I)
   A. Parathyroid neoplasia or hyperplasia (hyperparathyroidism)
   B. Pancreatic islet cell neoplasms (insulin, gastrin, VIP)
   C. Pituitary neoplasms (acromegaly, nonfunctioning tumors)
   D. Adrenal cortical neoplasms or hyperplasia (Cushing's syndrome)
   E. Thyroid involvement (hyperthyroidism; nonfunctional adenomas)
   F. About 2/3 of patients have adenomas of two or more systems
      and 1/5 develop adenoma in three or more systems
II. Multiple endocrine neoplasia type II (MEN II A)
   A. Pheochromocytoma
   B. Medullary carcinoma of the thyroid
   C. Parathyroid neoplasm or hyperplasia
III. Multiple endocrine neoplasia type III (MEN II B)
   A. Medullary carcinoma of the thyroid
   B. Pheochromocytoma
   C. Dysmorphic features (ganglioneuroma or neuromas of con-
      junctiva, buccal mucosa, tongue, larynx, gastrointestinal tract)

IV-47   RISK FACTORS PREDISPOSING
TO THROMBOSIS

I. Acquired
   A. Common
      1. Prior deep venous thrombosi
      2. Surgery with >30 minutes general anesthesia
      3. Surgery or trauma of pelvis or lower extremities
      4. Congestive heart failure
      5. Immobilization
      6. Malignancy
      7. Pregnancy
      8. Estrogen therapy
      9. Obesity
      10. Advanced age (>70)
   B. Uncommon
      1. Antiphospholipid antibody syndrome
      2. Nephrotic syndrome
      3. Inflammatory bowel disease
      4. Thrombocytosis
      5. Polycythemia vera
      6. Paroxysmal nocturnal hemoglobinuria
II. Inherited
   A. Antithrombin III deficiency
   B. Protein C deficiency
   C. Protein S deficiency
   D. Abnormal fibrogenics
   E. Abnormalities of plasma fibrinolytic system
   F. Homocystinuria
   C. Factor V Leiden mutation

From Senior IM et al (eds): *Cecil's textbook of medicine,* ed 20, Philadelphia, 1996, WB Saunders, p. 422.

CHAPTER V

Infectious Disease

V-1 DISEASE STATES CAUSING FEVER OF UNKNOWN ORIGIN (FUO)*

I. Infection
- A. Generalized
  1. Tuberculosis
  2. Histoplasmosis
  3. Typhoid fever
  4. CMV
  5. EB virus
  6. Miscellaneous: syphilis, brucellosis, toxoplasmosis, malaria
  7. HIV
- B. Localized
  1. Infective endocarditis
  2. Empyema
  3. Intraabdominal infection
     a. Peritonitis
     b. Cholangitis
     c. Abscess
  4. Urinary tract
     a. Pyelonephritis
     b. Perinephric abscess
     c. Prostatitis
  5. Decubitus ulcer
  6. Osteomyelitis
  7. Thrombophlebitis

II. Neoplasm
- A. Hematologic
  1. Lymphoma
  2. Hodgkin's disease
  3. Acute leukemia
- B. Tumors predisposed to cause fever
  1. Hepatoma
  2. Hypernephroma
  3. Atrial myxoma

Continued

V-1 DISEASE STATES CAUSING FEVER OF UNKNOWN ORIGIN (FUO)*—*cont'd*

III. Connective tissue disease
    A. RA, SLE
    B. Vasculitis
IV. Miscellaneous
    A. Drug induced
    B. Immune complex: SLE, RA
    C. Vasculitis
    D. Alcoholic liver disease
    E. Granulomatous hepatitis
    F. Inflammatory bowel disease, Whipple's disease
    G. Recurrent pulmonary emboli
    H. Factitious fever
    I. Undiagnosed

*Diagnostic criteria for FUO:
1. Illness of more than 3-weeks duration
2. Fever, intermittent or continuous
3. Documentation of fever >38.3° C
4. No obvious diagnosis after initial complete examination
Approximate current breakdown:
1. Neoplasms—7.0%
2. Infections—22.7%
3. Multisystem diseases—21.5%
4. Miscellaneous—14.5%
5. No diagnosis—25.6%
6. Drug-related—3%
7. Factitious—3.5%
8. Habitual hyperthermia—2.5%

From Knockaert DC et al: *Arch Intern Med* 152:51-55, 1992.

V-2 DIFFERENTIAL FOR THE ETIOLOGY OF PYOGENIC ABSCESS OF THE LIVER

  I. Cholangitis
      A. Choledocholithiasis
      B. Biliary tract tumors
      C. Pancreatic tumors
      D. Postsurgical strictures
 II. Direct extension from contiguous organs
      A. Lobar pneumonia
      B. Subphrenic abscess
      C. Pyelonephritis
      D. Perforated gastric ulcer
III. Embolization via portal venous system
      A. Appendicitis
      B. Diverticulitis
      C. Inflammatory bowel disease
      D. Proctitis
      E. Infected hemorrhoids
      F. Pancreatitis
      G. Splenitis
 IV. Embolization via hepatic artery
      A. Osteomyelitis
      B. Infective endocarditis
      C. Pneumonitis
  V. Trauma

V-3   CLINICAL FEATURES OF GENITOURINARY TUBERCULOSIS IN TWO SERIES OF PATIENTS

	Reference	
Clinical features	162	161
Number of patients	102	78
Primarily genitourinary symptoms	61%	71%
Back and flank pain	27%	10%
Dysuria, frequency, etc.	31%	34%
Constitutional symptoms	33%	14%
Abnormal urine, no symptoms	5%	20%
Abnormal urinalysis	66%	93%
Abnormal intravenous pyelogram	68%	93%
Tuberculin positive	88%	95%
Abnormal chest roentgenogram	75%	66%
Active pulmonary tuberculosis	38%	7%
Other old or active extrapulmonary disease	5%	20%
Urine culture positive		
For tuberculosis	80%	90%
For routine pathogens	45%	12%
Epididymitis/orchitis	19%	17%
Chronic prostatitis	6%	6%

From Haas DW, Des Prez RM. In Mandell GL, Bennett JE, Dolin R (eds): *Principles and practice of infectious disease,* ed 4, New York, 1995, Churchill Livingstone, p. 2237.

V-4   CRITERIA FOR THE DIAGNOSIS OF NONTUBERCULOSIS MYCOBACTERIAL DISEASE IN NON-IMMUNOCOMPROMISED HOSTS

I. The patient should have clinical evidence of disease compatible with the diagnosis
II. Isolation of the organism in colony counts of more than 100 on four or more occasions (with the exception of *M. kansasii)*
III. Isolation of the organism from ordinarily sterile sources
IV. Culture of the organism from a biopsy specimen
V. Check HIV status

From Davidson PT: *Clin Not Respir* 3-13, Summer 1979; Tellis CJ et al: *Med Clin North Am* 64(3):437, May 1980.

V-5   IMMUNOCOMPROMISED HOSTS

I. Hematologic malignancy (leukemia, lymphoma, multiple myeloma)
II. Solid tumors
III. Transplant recipients (renal, heart, heart-lung, liver, bone marrow)
IV. Corticosteroid therapy
V. Immunosuppressive agents
VI. Alcoholics
VII. Cirrhosis
VIII. Chronic renal failure
IX. Diabetes mellitus
X. Intravenous drug abusers
XI. Elderly
XII. AIDS
XIII. After splenectomy
XIV. Burns
XV. Malnutrition
XVI. Sickle cell anemia
XVII. Infants

V-6 PULMONARY INFECTIONS IN IMMUNOCOMPROMISED PATIENTS

I. Bacterial
  A. Pseudomonas
  B. Klebsiella
  C. Serratia
  D. Nocardia
  E. Tuberculosis
  F. Listeria
  G. *Escherichia coli*
  H. Enterobacter
  I. Staphylococcus
  J. Bacillus
  K. Clostridium
  L. Mycobacterium
  M. Legionella
  N. Salmonella
  O. *Streptococcus pneumoniae* (humoral deficiency)

II. Fungal
  A. Aspergillus
  B. Candida
  C. Coccidioidomycosis
  D. Cryptococcosis
  E. Phycomycetes
  F. Histoplasmosis
  G. Zygomycetes
  H. *Torulopsis glabrata*

III. Viral
  A. CMV
  B. Herpes simplex
  C. Varicella zoster
  D. Measles
  E. Adenovirus
  F. *Legionella pneumophila*
  G. Epstein-Barr virus

IV. Protozoa
  A. Pneumocystis
  B. Toxoplasma

V. Helminths
  A. *Strongyloides stercoralis*

From Matthay RA, Green WH: *Med Clin North Am* 64:534, 1980.

V-7 CLINICAL PULMONARY SYNDROMES OF HISTOPLASMOSIS
I. Primary pulmonary histoplasmosis
II. Acute histoplasmoma (unusually heavy exposure)
III. Disseminated histoplasmosis
IV. Chronic cavitating fibronodular histoplasmosis
V. Histoplasmosis
VI. Fibrosing mediastinitis

V-8 EXTRAPULMONARY MANIFESTATIONS OF *MYCOPLASMA PNEUMONIAE*
I. Hematologic
  A. Autoimmune hemolytic anemia
  B. Thrombocytopenia
  C. DIC
  D. Splenomegaly
II. Gastrointestinal
  A. Gastroenteritis
  B. Anicteric hepatitis
  C. Pancreatitis
III. Musculoskeletal
  A. Arthralgias
  B. Myalgias
  C. Polyarthritis
IV. Cardiac
  A. Pericarditis
  B. Myocarditis
  C. Conduction defects
  D. Pericardial effusion
V. Neurologic
  A. Meningitis
  B. Meningoencephalitis
  C. Transverse myelitis
  D. Peripheral and cranial neuropathies
  E. Cerebellar ataxia
VI. Dermatologic
  A. Erythema nodosum
  B. Erythema multiforme
  C. Stevens-Johnson syndrome
VII. Renal
  A. Interstitial nephritis
  B. Glomerulonephritis

From Murray HW, Tuazon C: *Med Clin North Am* 564:512, 1980.

V-9   EXTRAPULMONARY MANIFESTATIONS OF PSITTACOSIS

I. Cardiac
   A. Myocarditis
   B. Pericarditis
   C. Endocarditis
II. Neurologic
   A. Meningitis
   B. Encephalitis
   C. Seizure
III. Hematologic
   A. Anemia, nonhemolytic
   B. Hemolytic anemia
   C. DIC
   D. Splenomegaly
IV. Gastrointestinal
   A. Hepatitis
   B. Pancreatitis
V. Renal
   A. Nephritis
   B. Acute renal failure
   C. Proteinuria

From Murray HW, Tuazon C: *Med Clin North Am* 64:517, 1980.

V-10   EXTRAPULMONARY MANIFESTATIONS OF Q FEVER

I. Gastrointestinal
   A. Hepatitis
II. Cardiovascular
   A. Pericarditis
   B. Myocarditis
   C. Endocarditis
   D. Pericardial effusion
   E. Thrombophlebitis
   F. Arteritis
III. Ocular
   A. Uveitis
   B. Iritis
   C. Optic neuritis
IV. Neurologic
   A. Meningitis
   B. Peripheral neuropathy

From Murray HW, Tuazon C: *Med Clin North Am* 64:521, 1980.

V-11   FEATURES OF LEGIONELLA INFECTION

I. Pneumonia-bronchopneumonia with pleuritis; pleural effusion rare
- A. Fever: often high with rigors and chills >90%
- B. Nonproductive cough 90%
- C. Nausea/emesis
- D. Diarrhea with abdominal pain 30% to 50%
- E. Mental status changes 30%
  1. Lethargy
  2. Confusion
  3. Emotional lability
  4. Slurred speech
  5. Hallucination
  6. Seizures
  7. Coma
  8. Cerebellar dysfunction
  9. Peripheral neuropathy
  10. Motor weakness
- F. Myalgias
- G. Rash-macular
- H. Ocular-Roth and cotton wool exudates
- I. Laboratory: ↑ WBC, L shift
  - ↓Na, ↓ PO_4
  - ↑ AST, alk phos, LDH

II. Wound infection

III. Dialysis shunt infection

IV. Sinusitis

V. Pericarditis

Poor prognosticators: RR > 30, HR > 110, WBC > 14,000, Bands > 10%, renal failure, bilateral pulmonary involvement, hypoxemia.

From Meyer RD: *Rev Infect Dis* 5:258, 1983; Swartz MN: *Ann Intern Med* 90:492, 1979.

V-12 CLINICAL AND LABORATORY FEATURES OF CYTOMEGALOVIRUS MONONUCLEOSIS* (NON-IMMUNE COMPROMISED HOST)

Clinical	Estimated percent positive
I. Clinical	
A. Prolonged fever (>4 weeks)	20*
B. Hepatomegaly	30-50
C. Splenomegaly	30-50
D. Pharyngitis	5
E. Lymphadenopathy	10
II. Laboratory	
A. Lymphocytosis (>50% of cells)	98
B. Atypical lymphocytes (>20% of lymphocytes)	90
C. Rheumatoid factor, cryoglobulin	30
D. Cold agglutinin (anti-I or anti-i)	25
E. Antinuclear factor	20
F. Coombs' test	10
G. Fourfold CMV CF antibody change	85
H. Virus isolation:	
1. Urine	50-60
2. Saliva	70-80
I. Simultaneous infection with	
1. Epstein-Barr virus	5

*Fever of 2 weeks duration was the criterion for inclusion.
From Betts RF. In Stollerman GH (ed): *Advances in internal medicine,* vol 26, Chicago, 1980, Year Book Medical Publishers, Chicago, p. 455.

V-13 FACTORS ASSOCIATED WITH MORTALITY IN BRAIN ABSCESS

   I. Coma on admission
  II. Multiple brain abscesses
 III. Rupture of abscess in ventricle
  IV. Inaccurate or missed diagnosis
   V. Positive spinal fluid cultures
  VI. Brain abscess secondary to remote focus of infection
 VII. Absence of focal signs
VIII. Seizures
  IX. Symptoms of meningitis early in the illness

From Karandanis D, Shulman JA: *Arch Intern Med* 135:1145, 1975.

V-14   RISK FACTORS AFFECTING OUTCOME OF BACTEREMIA

   I. Male gender with age >75 years.
   II. Azotemia (creatinine >2.0 mg/dl)
   III. Pseudomonas species
   IV. *Streptococcus pneumoniae*
   V. Absence of fever (<38° C)
   VI. Coagulopathy
   VII. Interstitial pattern on chest x-ray involving more than half of both lung fields
   VIII. Delayed, inappropriate, or inadequate levels of antibiotics
   IX. Underlying immunosuppression
      A. Antecedent antimetabolites
      B. Antecedent corticosteroids
      C. Asplenia
      D. Diabetes mellitus
      E. Human immunodeficiency virus
   X. Lactic acidosis

From Kreger BE et al: *Am J Med* 68:344, 1980; Aube H et al: *Am J Med* 93:283, 1992.

V-15A MAJOR TYPES OF OSTEOMYELITIS*

Feature	Hematogenous	Secondary to contiguous focus of infection	Due to vascular insufficiency
I. Age distribution (yr)	Peaks at 1-20 and ≥50	≥50	>50
II. Bones involved	Long bones	Femur, tibia, skull, mandible	Feet
	Vertebrae		
III. Precipitating factors	Trauma (?)	Surgery	Diabetes mellitus
	Bacteremia	Soft-tissue infections	Peripheral vascular disease
IV. Bacteriology	Usually only one organism	Often mixed infection	Usually mixed infections
	S. aureus	*S. aureus*	*S. aureus* or *epidermidis*
	Gram-negative organisms	Gram-negative organisms	Streptococci
			Gram-negative organisms
		Anaerobic organisms	Anaerobic organisms
V. Episode	Initial	Initial	Inital and
Major clinical findings	Fever	Fever	Recurrent
	Local tenderness	Erythema	Pain
	Local swelling	Swelling	Swelling
	Limitation of motion	Heat	Erythema
			Drainage
			Ulceration
	Recurrent	Recurrent	
	Drainage	Drainage	
		Sinus	

From Norden CW. In Mandell GL, Douglas RG, Bennett JE (eds): *Principles and practice of infectious disease*, ed 3, New York, 1990, Churchill-Livingstone, pp. 922-930.

V-15B BACTERIOLOGY OF PROSTHETIC JOINT INFECTION

Pathogens	Frequency (%)
Staphylococci	53
S. epidermidis	28
S. aureus	25
Streptococci	20
B-Hemolytic streptococci	12
Viridans streptococci	8
Gram-negative aerobic bacilli	20
Anaerobes	7

From Brause BD. In Mandell GL, Douglas RG, Bennett JE (eds): *Principles and practice of infectious disease,* ed 3. New York, 1990, Churchill-Livingstone, p. 919.

V-16 SPECTRUM OF GONOCOCCAL INFECTIONS
   I. Urethritis
   II. Cervicitis
   III. Prostatitis
   IV. Epididymitis
   V. Pelvic inflammatory disease
   VI. Salpingitis
   VII. Proctitis
   VIII. Conjunctivitis
   IX. Pharyngitis
   X. Dermatitis
   XI. Arthritis
   XII. Perihepatitis
   XIII. Peritonitis
   XIV. Pericarditis
   XV. Myocarditis
   XVI. Endocarditis
   XVII. Hepatitis
   XVIII. Meningitis
   XIX. Osteomyelitis
   XX. Sepsis (Waterhouse-Friedrichson Syndrome)
   XXI. Disseminated gonococcal infection ("arthritis-dermatitis syndrome")

V-17   CLINICAL FEATURES OF FOOD POISONING SECONDARY TO BOTULISM: SYMPTOMS AND SIGNS IN PATIENTS WITH THE COMMON TYPE OF HUMAN BOTULISM

	Type A (%)	Type B (%)	Type E (%)
Neurologic symptoms			
Dysphagia	96	97	82
Dry mouth	83	100	93
Diplopia	90	92	39
Dysarthria	100	69	50
Upper extremity weakness	86	64	NA
Lower extremity weakness	76	64	NA
Blurred vision	100	42	91
Dyspnea	91	34	88
Paresthesia	20	12	NA
Gastrointestinal symptoms			
Constipation	73	73	52
Nausea	73	57	84
Vomiting	70	50	96
Abdominal cramps	33	46	NA
Diarrhea	35	8	39
Miscellaneous			
Fatigue	92	69	84
Sore throat	75	39	38
Dizziness	86	30	63
Neurologic findings			
Ptosis	96	55	46
Diminished gag reflex	81	54	NA
Ophthalmoparesis	87	46	NA
Facial paresis	84	48	NA
Tongue weakness	91	31	66
Pupils fixed or dilated	33	56	75
Nystagmus	44	4	NA
Upper extremity weakness	91	62	NA
Lower extremity weakness	82	59	NA
Ataxia	24	13	NA
DTR's diminished or absent	54	29	NA
DTR's hyperactive	12	0	NA
Initial mental status			
Alert	88	93	27
Lethargic	4	4	73
Obtunded	8	4	0

From Bleck TP. In Mandell GL, Bennett JE, Dolin R (eds): *Principles and practice of infectious disease*, ed 4, New York, 1995, Churchill Livingstone, p. 2180.

V-18   ANTIBIOTIC ASSOCIATED PSEUDOMEMBRANOUS COLITIS

I. Antibiotics implicated
   A. Lincomycin
   *B. Amoxicillin
   C. Erythromycin
   D. Neomycin
   *E. Clindamycin
   *F. Cephalosporins
   G. Oral penicillin
   H. Vancomycin
   *I. Ampicillin
   J. Tetracycline
   K. Gentamicin
   L. Sulfamethoxazole/trimethoprim
   M. Quinolones
II. Clinical features
   A. Diarrhea (rarely bloody)
   B. Crampy abdominal pain and tenderness to palpation
   C. Fever
   D. Toxic megacolon (rare)
   E. Leukocytosis
III. Diagnosis
   A. Pseudomembranous lesion (plaques)visualized at sigmoid-oscopy (75% to 80% of cases)
   B. Demonstration of *Clostridium difficile* toxin
IV. Treatment
   A. Discontinue antibiotics
   B. Metronidazole or vancomycin–10% to 15% of patients relapse after treatment
   C. Bile salt sequestering agents (cholestyramine)

*Especially important.

V-19 TOXIC SHOCK SYNDROME

I. Etiology and epidemiology
- A. Approximately 50% of cases occur in women <30 years of age
- B. 50% of cases not associated with menstruation (⅓ are men)
  1. Drug abusers
  2. Homosexuals
  3. Staphylococcal/streptococcal sepsis
  4. Surgical wound infections
  5. Nonsurgical traumatic wounds
  6. Parturition
  7. Staphylococcal/streptococcal pneumonia
- C. Strong correlation between toxic shock syndrome and recovery of *Staphylococcus aureus* from vaginal cultures
- D. Toxins elaborated by *S. aureus* (TSST-1) and group A streptococcus exotoxin A are responsible for the clinical manifestations

II. Clinical features
- A. Multisystem disease
  1. Rash—macular, erythematous, often desquamative
  2. Fever
  3. Hypotension
  4. Desquamation—1 to 2 weeks after illness onset, particularly of palms and soles
  5. Volume depletion
  6. Renal insufficiency
  7. Liver test abnormalities
  8. Nausea, vomiting, diarrhea
  9. Thrombocytopenia, subclinical DIC
  10. Disorientation with/without focal neurologic signs
  11. Mucous membranes—hyperemia
- B. Diagnosis
  1. No. 1-4 and any 3 of items no. 5-11 or no. 1-3 and any 5 of items no. 5-11

III. Differential diagnosis
- A. Meningococcemia
- B. Rocky Mountain spotted fever
- C. Leptospirosis
- D. Drug eruption
- E. Rubella

From Bone RC, Barkoviak J: *J Crit Illness* 7(7):1032-1044, 1992.

V-20 ANAEROBIC INFECTIONS

I. Host factors that may predispose to development of anaerobic infection
   A. Disruption of normal cutaneous or mucosal barriers
   B. Tissue injury (accidental trauma, surgery, or invasive diagnostic procedure)
   C. Impaired blood supply (including microvascular disease)
   D. Tissue necrosis
   E. Obstruction of hollow viscus (tracheobronchial tree, biliary tract, gastrointestinal tract, fallopian tube)
   F. Presence of foreign body
   G. Underlying malignancy

II. Clinical clues to anaerobic infections
   A. Foul order of lesion or discharge
   B. Location of infection in proximity to mucosal surface
   C. Tissue necrosis; abscess formation
   D. Infection secondary to human or animal bite
   E. Gas in tissues or discharges
   F. Classical clinical picture such as gas gangrene
   G. Previous therapy with aminoglycoside antibiotics (e.g., neomycin, gentamicin, and amikacin)
   H. Black discoloration or red fluorescence under UV light of blood containing exudates (pigmented *Bacteroides* infection)
   I. Septic thrombophlebitis
   J. Presence of "sulfur granules" in discharges (actinomycosis)
   K. Unique morphology on Gram stain of exudate (pleomorphic or otherwise distinctive)
   L. Failure of culture to grow aerobically, organisms seen on Gram stain of original exudate

III. Source of anaerobic bacteremia by portal of entry (n = 40)
   A. Gastrointestinal tract–60%
   B. Skin–15%
   C. Genitourinary tract–8%
   D. Oral–2%
   E. Uncertain–13%

From Finegold SM, George WL, Mulligan ME. Anaerobic infections. In Cotsonas NJ (ed): *Disease-a-Month*, ed 31, Chicago, 1985, Year Book Medical Publishers, pp. 21, 26; Lombardi DP, Engleberg NC: *Am J Med 92:53-60, 1992.*

V-21 *LISTERIA MONOCYTOGENES INFECTIONS*

   I. Presentations
- A. Meningoencephalitis
- B. Septicemia
- C. Endocarditis
- D. Endophthalmitis
- E. Peritonitis
- F. Pleurisy
- G. Osteomyelitis
- H. Lymphadenitis
- I. Conjunctivitis
- J. Cholecystitis
- K. Visceral abscesses
- L. Amnionitis

  II. Predisposing factors
- A. Malignancy
- B. Immunosuppression
- C. Alcoholism
- D. Diabetes
- E. Chronic hepatic disease
- F. Pregnancy
- G. AIDS

From Nieman RE, Lorber B: *Rev Infectious Dis* 2:207, 1980; Morbidity & Mortality Weekly Reports: Centers for Disease Control 31:207, 513, 1991.

V-22   EFFECTIVE DRUG REGIMENS FOR THE INITIAL TREATMENT OF TUBERCULOSIS*

I. Daily isoniazid, rifampin, and pyrazinamide for 8 weeks followed by 16 weeks of isoniazid and rifampin daily or 2 to 3 times per week.* (In areas where the isoniazid resistance rate is not documented to be less than 4%, ethambutol or streptomycin should be added to the initial regimen until susceptibility to isoniazid and rifampin is demonstrated.)

II. Daily isoniazid, rifampin, pyrazinamide, and streptomycin or ethambutol for 2 weeks followed by 2 times per week administration of the same drugs for 6 weeks, and subsequently with 2 times per week administration of isoniazid and rifampin for 16 weeks.*

III. Treat by directly observed therapy (DOT) 3 times per week with isoniazid, rifampin, pyrazinamide, and ethambutol or streptomycin for 6 months.

*All regimens administered 2 times per week or 3 times per week should be monitored by DOT for the duration of therapy.

From *Am J Respir Crit Care Med:* 149:1359-1374, 1994.

V-23 MANIFESTATIONS OF LYME DISEASE BY STAGE*

	Localized (Stage I)	Early infection disseminated (Stage II)	Late infection persistent (Stage III)
I. Skin†	Erythema migrans	Secondary annular lesions, malar rash, diffuse erythema or urticaria, evanescent lesions, lymphocytoma	Acrodermatitis chronica atrophicans, localized scleroderma-like lesions
II. Musculoskeletal system		Migratory pain in joints, tendons, bursae, muscle, bone; brief arthritis attacks; myositis‡; osteomyelitis‡; panniculitis‡	Prolonged arthritis attacks, chronic arthritis, peripheral enthesopathy, periostitis or joint subluxations below lesions of acrodermatitis
III. Neurologic system		Meningitis, cranial neuritis, Bell's palsy, motor or sensory radiculoneuritis, subtle encephalitis, mononeuritis multiplex, myelitis‡ chorea‡, cerebellar ataxia‡	Chronic encephalomyelitis, spastic parapareses, ataxic gait, subtle mental disorders, chronic axonal polyradiculopathy, lopathy, dementia‡
IV. Lymphatic system	Regional lymphadenopathy	Regional or generalized lymphadenopathy, splenomegaly	

V. Heart	Atrioventricular nodal block, myopericarditis, pancarditis
VI. Eyes	Conjunctivitis, iritis‡, choroiditis‡, retinal hemorrhage or detachment‡, panophthalmitis‡ Keratitis
VII. Liver	Mild or recurrent hepatitis
VIII. Respiratory system	Nonexudative sore throat, nonproductive cough, adult respiratory distress syndrome†
IX. Kidney	Microscopic hematuria or proteinuria
X. Genitourinary system	Orchitis‡
XI. Constitutional minor symptoms	Severe malaise and fatigue Fatigue

*The classification by stages provides a guideline for the expected timing of the illness's manifestations but this may vary from case to case.
†Systems are listed from the most to the least commonly affected.
‡The inclusion of this manifestation is based on one or a few cases.
From Steere AC: *N Engl J Med* 321(9):586-596, 1989.

V-24 CHRONIC FATIGUE SYNDROME: DIAGNOSTIC CRITERIA*

I. Major criteria
1. New onset of persistent or relapsing, debilitating fatigue, or easy fatigability in a person who has no previous history of similar symptoms, that does not resolve with bedrest, and that is severe enough to reduce or impair average daily activity below 50% of the patient's premorbid activity level for a period of at least 6 months.
2. Other clinical conditions that may produce similar symptoms must be excluded by thorough evaluation based on history, physical examination and appropriate laboratory findings.

II. Minor criteria
A. Symptom Criteria
1. Mild fever (oral temperature between 37.5 and 38.6° C, if measured by the patient) or chills
2. Sore throat
3. Painful lymph nodes in the anterior or posterior cervical or axillary distribution
4. Unexplained generalized muscle weakness
5. Muscle discomfort or myalgia
6. Prolonged generalized fatigue after levels of exercise that would have been easily tolerated in the patient premorbid state
7. Generalized headaches
8. Migratory arthralgia without joint swelling or redness
9. Neuropsychologic complaints including
   a. Photophobia
   b. Transient visual scotomata
   c. Forgetfulness
   d. Excessive irritability
   e. Confusion
   f. Difficulty thinking
   g. Inability to concentrate
   h. Depression
10. Sleep disturbance (hypersomnia or insomnia)
11. Description of the initial symptom complex as initially developing over a period of a few hours to a few days
B. Physical criteria
1. Low grade fever (oral temperature between 37.6 and 38.6° C or rectal temperature between 37.8 and 38.8° C)
2. Nonexudative pharyngitis
3. Palpable or tender anterior or posterior cervical or axillary lymph nodes.
   (Note: lymph nodes greater than 2 cm in diameter suggest other causes)

*To make the diagnosis of chronic fatigue syndrome, both of the major criteria must be present. In addition, patients must exhibit at least 6 of the 11 symptom criteria and at least 2 of the 3 physical criteria, or 8 or more of the symptom criteria.

From Schooley RT. In Mandell GL, Bennett JE, Dolin R (eds): *Principles and practice of infectious disease,* ed 4, New York, 1995, Churchill Livingstone, p. 1306.

CHAPTER VI

Nephrology

VI-1   DIFFERENTIAL DIAGNOSIS OF METABOLIC ALKALOSIS

  I. Sodium chloride-responsive (U_{Cl} <10 mmoles per liter)
   A. Gastrointestinal disorders:
      1. Vomiting
      2. Gastric drainage
      3. Vilous adenoma of the colon
      4. Chloride diarrhea
   B. Diuretic therapy
   C. Rapid correction of chronic hypercapnia
   D. Cystic fibrosis
 II. Sodium chloride-resistant (U_{Cl} >20 mmoles per liter)
   A. Excess mineralocorticoid activity
      1. Hyperaldosteronism
      2. Cushing's syndrome
      3. Bartter's syndrome
      4. Excess licorice intake
   B. Profound potassium depletion
III. Unclassified
   A. Alkali administration
   B. Milk-alkali syndrome
   C. Nonparathyroid hypercalcemia
   D. Massive transfusion
   E. Glucose ingestion after starvation
   F. Large doses of carbenicillin or penicillin
   G. Recovery from organic acidosis
   H. Antacids and exchange resins in renal failure

From Kaehny WD, Shapiro JI. In Schrier RW (ed): *Renal and electrolyte disorders,* ed 4, Boston, 1992, Little, Brown, p. 198.

VI-2   DIFFERENTIAL DIAGNOSIS OF METABOLIC ACIDOSIS WITH INCREASED ANION GAP

I. Increased Acid Production
   A. Diabetic ketoacidosis
   B. Alcoholic ketoacidosis
   C. Starvation ketoacidosis
   D. Lactic acidosis
      1. Secondary to hypotension, hypovolemia, hypoxemia
      2. Secondary to drugs and toxins
      3. Enzyme defects
   E. Poisons and drug toxicity
      1. Salicylates
      2. Methanol
      3. Ethylene glycol
      4. Paraldehyde
   F. Hyperosmolar hyperglycemic nonketotic coma
II. Renal failure
   A. Acute renal failure
   B. Chronic renal failure

From Levinsky NG. In Isselbacher KJ et al (eds): *Harrison's principles of internal medicine*, ed 13, New York, 1994, McGraw-Hill, p. 256.

VI-3 DIFFERENTIAL DIAGNOSIS OF METABOLIC ACIDOSIS WITH NORMAL ANION GAP (HYPERCHLOREMIC ACIDOSIS)

I. Renal tubular acidosis
II. Uremic acidosis (early)
III. Intestinal loss of bicarbonate or organic acid anions
    A. Diarrhea
    B. Pancreatic fistula
IV. Ureteroenterostomy
V. Drugs
    A. Acetazolamide
    B. Sulfamylon
    C. Cholestyramine
    D. Acidifying agents: NH_4Cl, oral $CaCl_2$, arginine-HCl, lysine-HCl
    E. Aldactone (in patients with cirrhosis)
VI. Rapid IV hydration
VII. Correction of respiratory alkalosis
VIII. Hyperalimentation

From Emmett M, Narins RG: *Medicine* 56:38, 1977.

VI-4 DIFFERENTIAL DIAGNOSIS OF A LOW ANION GAP

I. Reduced concentration of unmeasured anions
    A. Dilution
    B. Hypoalbuminemia
II. Increased unmeasured cations
    A. Paraproteinemia
    B. Hypercalcemia, hypermagnesemia, trimethane (tris buffer), lithium toxicity
III. Laboratory error
    A. Systemic error:
        1. Underestimation of serum sodium secondary to severe hypernatremia or hyperviscosity
        2. Bromism
    B. Random error: falsely decreased serum sodium, falsely increased serum chloride or bicarbonate

From Oh MS, Carroll HG: *N Engl J Med* 297:814, 1977; Emmett M, Narrins RG: *Medicine* 56:38, 1977.

VI-5 DIFFERENTIAL DIAGNOSIS OF HYPOKALEMIA

I. Inadequate dietary intake
II. Gastrointestinal losses
   A. Vomiting
   B. Diarrhea
   C. Chronic laxative abuse
III. Renal losses
   A. Diuretics
   B. Mineralocorticoid excess
      1. Primary aldosteronism
         a. adenoma
         b. bilateral adrenal hyperplasia
      2. Cushing's syndrome
         a. primary adrenal disease
         b. secondary to non-endocrine tumor
      3. Accelerated hypertension
      4. Renal vascular hypertension
      5. Renin producing tumor
      6. Adrenogenital syndrome
      7. Licorice excess
   C. Bartter's syndrome
   D. Liddle's syndrome
   E. Renal tubular acidosis
   F. Metabolic alkalosis
   G. Acute hyperventilation
   H. Starvation
   I. Ureterosigmoidostomy
   J. Antibiotics—carbenicillin, amphotericin, gentamicin
   K. Diabetic ketoacidosis
   L. Acute leukemia
IV. Cellular shift
   A. Alkalosis
   B. Periodic paralysis
   C. Barium poisoning
   D. Insulin administration

From Kunau RT, Stein JH: *Clin Nephrol* 7:173, 1977.

VI-6   DIFFERENTIAL DIAGNOSIS OF HYPERKALEMIA

I. Pseudohyperkalemia
   A. Improper collection of blood
   B. Hematologic disorders with increased white blood cells or platelets counts
II. Exogenous potassium load
   A. Oral or intravenous KCl
   B. Potassium containing drugs
   C. Transfusion
III. Cellular shift of potassium
   A. Tissue damage–trauma, burns, rhabdomyolysis
   B. Destruction of tumor tissue
   C. Drugs
      1. Digitalis overdose
      2. Arginine infusion
      3. Succinylcholine
      4. Alpha-adrenergic agonists
      5. Beta-adrenergic antagonists
   D. Acidosis
   E. Hyperkalemic periodic paralysis
   F. Hyperosmolality
IV. Decreased renal potassium excretion
   A. Acute renal failure
   B. Chronic renal failure
   C. Drugs
      1. Potassium sparing diuretics
      2. Heparin therapy
      3. NSAIDs
      4. Cyclosporine
      5. Pentamidine
      6. FK 506
      7. Angiotensin converting enzyme inhibitors
   D. Mineralocorticoid deficiency
      1. Addison's disease
      2. Bilateral adrenalectomy
      3. Hypoaldosteronism
         a. Hyporeninemic hypoaldosteronism
         b. Specific enzyme defect
         c. Tubular unresponsiveness
   E. Congenital adrenal hyperplasia
   F. Primary defect in potassium transport

From Kunau RT, Stein JH: *Clin Nephrol* 7:173, 1977.

VI-7   CAUSES OF HYPERNATREMIA

I. Euvolemic hypernatremia (pure water loss)
   A. Extrarenal losses
      1. Respiratory (tachypnea)
      2. Dermal (sweating, fever)
   B. Renal losses
      1. Central diabetes insipidus
      2. Nephrogenic diabetes insipidus
   C. Other
      1. Inability to gain access to fluids
      2. Hypodipsia or adipsia
      3. Reset osmostat? (essential hypernatremia)
II. Hypovolemic hypernatremia (water deficit in excess of sodium deficit)
   A. Extrarenal losses
      1. Gastrointestinal losses (e.g., diarrhea, vomiting, fistulas)
      2. Dermal (burns, excessive sweating)
   B. Renal losses
      1. Osmotic diuresis (mannitol, glucose, urea)
      2. Loop diuretics
      3. Postobstructive diuresis
      4. Intrinsic renal disease
      5. Acute renal failure, diuretic phase
III. Hypervolemic hypernatremia (sodium gain in excess of water gain)
   A. Hypertonic saline or HaHCO3 administration
   B. Infants or comatose patients given hypertonic feedings
   C. Mineralocorticoid excess
      1. Cushing's syndrome
      2. Primary hyperaldosteronism

From Lanese DM, Teitelbaum I. In Jacobson HR, Striker GE, Klahr S (eds): *The principles and practice of nephrology,* ed 2, St Louis, 1995, Mosby, p. 894.

VI-8   DIFFERENTIAL DIAGNOSIS OF HYPONATREMIA

I. Extracellular fluid-volume depleted
   A. Renal losses
      1. Diuretics
      2. Adrenal insufficiency
      3. Salt losing nephropathy
      4. Renal tubular acidosis with bicarbonaturia
      5. Osmotic diuresis (glucose, mannitol, urea)
   B. Extra-renal losses
      1. Vomiting
      2. Diarrhea
      3. "3rd space" (e.g. burns, pancreatitis, traumatized muscle)
II. Extracellular fluid–normal or modest excess
   A. Hypothyroidism
   B. Syndrome of inappropriate ADH secretion
   C. Pain, emotion, drugs
   D. Glucocorticoid deficiency
III. Extracellular fluid-profound excess (edema)
   A. Nephrotic syndrome
   B. Cirrhosis
   C. Congestive heart failure
   D. Renal failure (acute and chronic)
IV. Artifactual
   A. Laboratory error
   B. Hyperglycemia, hypertriglyceridemia, hyperproteinemia

From Schrier RW, Berl T. In Schrier RW (ed): *Renal and electrolyte disorders,* ed 4, Boston, 1992, Little, Brown, p. 52.

VI-9 DIFFERENTIAL DIAGNOSIS OF RENAL TUBULAR ACIDOSIS (RTA) TYPE I (DISTAL)

I. Primary
   A. Idiopathic
   B. Genetic
II. Genetically transmitted systemic diseases
   A. Marfan's syndrome
   B. Sickle cell anemia
   C. Carbonic anhydrase I deficiency
   D. Galactosemia
   E. Hereditary fructose intolerance
   F. Ehlers-Danlos syndrome
   G. Fabry's disease
   H. Hereditary elliptocytosis
III. Metabolic disorders
   A. Idiopathic hypercalciuria–sporadic and hereditary
   B. Hyperthyroidism
   C. Primary hyperparathyroidism
   D. Vitamin D intoxication
   E. Mineralocorticoid deficiency
IV. Hypergammaglobulinemic disorders
   A. Amyloidosis
   B. Idiopathic hyperglobulinemia
   C. Hyperglobulinemic purpura
   D. Cryoglobulinemia
V. Medullary sponge kidney
VI. Hepatic cirrhosis
VII. Wilson's disease
VIII. Drug induced
   A. Amphotericin B
   B. Vitamin D
   C. Lithium
   D. Toluene
   E. Cyclamate
   F. Analgesics
   G. Amiloride
   H. Glue
   I. Balkan nephropathy
IX. Pyelonephritis
X. Leprosy
XI. Renal transplantation

Continued

VI-9   DIFFERENTIAL DIAGNOSIS OF RENAL TUBULAR ACIDOSIS (RTA) TYPE I (DISTAL)—*cont'd*

XII. Obstructive nephropathy
XIII. Autoimmune disorders
    A. Sjögren's syndrome
    B. Thyroiditis
    C. Pulmonary fibrosis
    D. Primary biliary cirrhosis
    E. Systemic lupus erythematosus
    F. Chronic active hepatitis
XIV. Multiple myeloma
XV.   Hodgkin's disease

From Sebastian A, McSherry E, Morris R. In Brenner B, Rector F (eds): *The kidney*, vol I, Philadelphia, 1986, WB Saunders, p. 482.

VI-10   DIFFERENTIAL DIAGNOSIS OF RENAL TUBULAR ACIDOSIS (RTA) TYPE II (PROXIMAL)

I. Primary
    A. Sporadic
    B. Genetic-Fanconi's syndrome
II. Inborn errors of metabolism
    A. Wilson's disease
    B. Cystinosis
    C. Others: Tyrosinosis, Lowe's syndrome, hereditary fructose intolerance, pyruvate carboxylase deficiency, galactosemia, glycogen storage disease (Type II)
III. Metabolic disorders
    A. Vitamin D deficiency
    B. Primary or secondary hyperparathyroidism
    C. Pseudo-vitamin D deficiency
IV. Disorders of protein metabolism
    A. Nephrotic syndrome
    B. Multiple myeloma
    C. Sjögren's syndrome
    D. Amyloidosis
    E. Other dysproteinemias
V. Medullary cystic disease
VI. Renal transplantation
VII. Drugs: outdated tetracycline, 6-mercaptopurine, streptozotocin, toluene, sulfonamide, sulfamylon, acetazolamide
VIII. Heavy metals: lead, cadmium, mercury

VI-11 DIFFERENTIAL DIAGNOSIS OF RENAL TUBULAR ACIDOSIS (RTA) TYPE IV

I. Aldosterone deficiency
   A. Combined deficiency of aldosterone and adrenal glucocorticoid hormones
      1. Addison's disease
      2. Bilateral adrenalectomy
      3. Inherited impairment of steroidogenesis: 21-hydroxylase deficiency ("congenital adrenal hyperplasia")
   B. Selective deficiency of aldosterone
      1. Inherited impairment of aldosterone biosynthesis: corticosterone methyl oxidase deficiency
      2. Secondary to deficient renin secretion
         a. Diabetic nephropathy
         b. Chronic tubulointerstitial disease with glomerular insufficiency
         c. Indomethacin administration
      3. Chronic idiopathic hypoaldosteronism in adults and children

II. Pseudohypoaldosteronism (attenuated renal response to aldosterone with secondary hyperreninemia and hyperaldosteronism)
   A. Classic pseudohypoaldosteronism of infancy
   B. Chronic tubulo-interstitial disease with glomerular insufficiency "salt-wasting nephritis"
   C. Drugs: spironolactone; amiloride; triamterene

III. Attenuated renal response to aldosterone + aldosterone deficiency
   A. Selective tubule dysfunction with impaired renin secretion
   B. Chronic tubulo-interstitial disease with glomerular insufficiency
      1. Associated deficient renin secretion
      2. Renin status uncertain
   C. Renal transplantation with deficient renin secretion
   D. Lupus nephritis with deficient renin secretion

IV. Uncertain pathophysiology
   A. Chronic pyelonephritis
   B. Lupus nephritis
   C. Renal transplantation
   D. Acute glomerulonephritis
   E. Renal amyloidosis

From Sebastian A et al: *Am J Med* 72:301, 1982.

VI-12 CAUSES OF ACUTE RENAL FAILURE

I. Prerenal failure
   A. Decreased cardiac output
      1. Myocardial infarction
      2. Cardiac dysrhythmia
      3. Decompensated congestive heart failure
      4. Cardiac tamponade
      5. Pulmonary embolism
      6. Positive-pressure mechanical ventilation
   B. Hypovolemia with or without hypotension
      1. Decreased intake
      2. External losses of extracellular fluid
         a. Renal losses
         b. Gastrointestinal losses
         c. Dermal losses
   C. Internal losses, redistribution, or third spacing
      1. Hypoalbuminemia
      2. Liver cirrhosis
      3. Nephrotic syndrome
      4. Pancreatitis
      5. Traumatized tissues
      6. Peritonitis
      7. Intestinal obstruction
      8. Burns
   D. Peripheral vasodilation
      1. Sepsis
      2. Shock
      3. Liver failure
      4. Antihypertensive agents
      5. Drug overdose
   E. Renal vascular occlusion or severe constriction
      1. Atherosclerosis
      2. Embolism
      3. Thrombosis
      4. Vasculitis
      5. Renal pedicle compression
      6. Dissection of abdominal aortic aneurysm
      7. Endotoxin
      8. Cyclosporine
   F. Disruption in renal autoregulation
      1. Prostaglandin inhibitors
      2. Angiotensin-converting enzyme inhibitors

Continued

VI-12 CAUSES OF ACUTE RENAL FAILURE—*cont'd*

II. Intrinsic renal failure
- A. Vascular diseases
  1. Malignant hypertension
  2. Vasculitis
  3. Hemolytic-uremic syndrome
  4. Thrombotic thrombocytopenic purpura
  5. Preeclampsia
  6. Postpartum nephrosclerosis
  7. Cholesterol emboli
  8. Renal cortical necrosis
- B. Glomerular diseases
  1. Acute postinfectious glomerulonephritis
  2. Goodpasture's syndrome
  3. Rapidly progressive glomerulonephritis
  4. Lupus nephritis
  5. IgA nephropathy
  6. Interstitial nephritis
- C. Interstitial nephritis
  1. Infectious causes (bacteria, fungi, viruses, and so on)
  2. Infiltrative causes (lymphoma, sarcoidosis, and so on)
  3. Related to drugs
  4. Idiopathic
- D. Tubular diseases—"acute tubular necrosis"
  1. Ischemic injury
  2. Prolonged prerenal azotemia
  3. Shock, postoperative
  4. Crush syndrome, major trauma
- E. Nephrotoxic injury (refer to table VI-14)
- F. Pigment injury (myoglobinuria, hemoglobinuria)
- G. Crystal-induced injury
  1. Uric acid nephropathy
  2. Oxalate nephropathy
  3. Sulfadiazine
  4. Acyclovir
  5. Methotrexate

Continued

VI-12   CAUSES OF ACUTE RENAL FAILURE—*cont'd*

  H. Metabolic causes
    1. Hypercalcemia
    2. Myeloma proteins
    3. Light-chain nephropathy
III. Post-renal failure
  A. Intraureteral obstruction
    1. Blood clots
    2. Stones
    3. Papillary necrosis
    4. Fungus balls
  B. Extraureteral obstruction
    1. Aberrant vessels
    2. Ligation
    3. Malignancy
    4. Endometriosis
    5. Retroperitoneal fibrosis, tumors
  C. Lower urinary tract obstruction
    1. Urethral stricture
    2. Prostatic hypertrophy or cancer
    3. Bladder cancer
    4. Cervical cancer
    5. Neurogenic bladder

From Cadnapaphornchai P, Alavalapati RK, McDonald FD. In Jacobson HR, Striker GE, Klahr S (eds): *The principles and practice of nephrology,* ed 2, St Louis, 1995, Mosby, p. 556.

VI-13 DIFFERENTIAL DIAGNOSIS OF COMMON MECHANICAL CAUSES OF URINARY TRACT OBSTRUCTION

Ureter*	Bladder outlet†	Urethra†
CONGENITAL		
Ureteropelvic junction narrowing or obstruction	Bladder neck obstruction	Posterior urethral valves
	Ureterocele	Anterior urethral valves
Ureterovesical junction narrowing or obstruction		Stricture
		Meatal stenosis
Ureterocele		Phimosis
Retrocaval ureter		
ACQUIRED INTRINSIC DEFECTS		
Calculi	Benign prostatic hypertrophy	Stricture
Inflammation		Tumor
Trauma	Cancer of prostate	Calculi
Sloughed papillae	Cancer of bladder	Trauma
Tumor	Calculi	Phimosis
Blood clots	Diabetic neuropathy	
Uric acid crystals	Spinal cord disease	
	Anticholinergic drugs and alpha-adrenergic antagonists	
ACQUIRED EXTRINSIC DEFECTS		
Pregnant uterus	Carcinoma of cervix, colon	Trauma
Retroperitoneal fibrosis		
Aortic aneurysm	Trauma	
Uterine leiomyomata		
Carcinoma of uterus, prostate, bladder, colon, rectum		
Retroperitoneal lymphoma		
Accidental surgical ligation		

*Lesions are typically associated with unilateral obstruction.
†Lesions are typically associated with bilateral obstruction.
From Brenner BM, Seifter JL. In Isselbacher KJ et al (eds): *Harrison's principles of internal medicine,* ed 13, New York, 1994, McGraw-Hill, p. 1333.

VI-14   MAJOR NEPHROTOXINS

I. Exogenous
   A. Metals (Hg, Au, Ag, Ar, Pb, Cd, Ur, Li)
   B. Solvents (halogenated hydrocarbons)
   C. Diagnostic agents (contrast agents)
   D. Therapeutic agents
      1. Antibiotics (aminoglycosides, amphotericin B, sulfas, tetraycylines, penicillins, pentamidine, foscarnet)
      2. Analgesics (phenacetin, ASA, NSAIDs)
      3. Anesthetics (methoxyflurane)
      4. Hormones (vitamin D)
      5. Antineoplastics (methotrexate, cis-platinum, cyclophosphamide)
      6. Radiation
      7. Immunosuppressive Agents (cyclosporine)
   E. Miscellaneous (venoms, mushrooms, fluoride, ethylene glycol)
II. Endogenous
   A. Uric acid
   B. Oxalate
   C. Pigments (myoglobin, hemoglobin)
   D. Light chain disease
   E. Hormones (PTH)
   F. Calcium

VI-15 DIFFERENTIATION OF DEHYDRATION AND ACUTE TUBULAR INJURY AS A CAUSE OF OLIGURIA

	U_{osm} (mEq)	U_{Na}	U/P creatinine	Renal failure index $\dfrac{U_{Na}}{U/P\ creatinine}$	Fractional excretion Na $\dfrac{U/P_{Na}}{U/P\ creatinine} \times 100$	Response to fluid challenge with increased urine output
Dehydration	>500	<20	>40:1	<1	<1	(+)
Acute tubular necrosis	<350	>40	<20:1	>1	>1	(−)

VI-16 DIFFERENTIAL DIAGNOSIS OF ACUTE GLOMERULONEPHRITIS

I. Infectious diseases
   A. Poststreptococcal glomerulonephritis
   B. Nonpoststreptococcal glomerulonephritis
      1. Bacterial: infective endocarditis, "shunt nephritis," sepsis, pneumococcal pneumonia, typhoid fever, secondary syphilis, meningococcemia
      2. Viral: Hepatitis B, infectious mononucleosis, mumps, measles, varicella, vaccinia, echovirus, and coxsackievirus
      3. Parasitic: Malaria, toxoplasmosis
II. Multisystem diseases: Systemic lupus erythematosus, vasculitis, Schönlein-Henoch purpura, Goodpasture's syndrome
III. Primary glomerular diseases: Membranoproliferative glomerulonephritis, Berger's disease, "pure" mesangial proliferative glomerulonephritis
IV. Miscellaneous; Guillain-Barré syndrome, irradiation of Wilms' tumor, self-administered diphtheria-pertussis-tetanus vaccine, serum sickness

From Glasslock RJ, Brenner BM. In Isselbacher KJ et al (eds): *Harrison's principles of internal medicine*, ed 13, New York, 1994, McGraw-Hill, p. 1295.

VI-17 DIFFERENTIAL DIAGNOSIS OF THE NEPHROTIC SYNDROME

I. Primary glomerular disease
   A. Minimal change disease
   B. Focal and segmental glomerulosclerosis
   C. Mesangial proliferative glomerulonephritis
   D. Membranous glomerulopathy
   E. Membranoproliferative glomerulonephritis
   F. Other uncommon lesions
      1. Crescenteric glomerulonephritis
      2. Focal and segmental proliferative glomerulonephritis
      3. Fibrillary and/or immunotactoid glomerulonephritis
II. Secondary to other diseases
   A. Infections
      1. Poststreptococcal glomerulonephritis
      2. Endocarditis
      3. Hepatitis B
      4. Syphilis
      5. Leprosy
      6. "Shunt nephritis"
      7. Infectious mononucleosis
      8. Malaria
      9. Schistosomiasis
      10. Filariasis
      11. AIDS
   B. Drugs
      1. Gold
      2. Mercury
      3. Penicillamine
      4. Heroin
      5. Probenecid
      6. Captopril
      7. Antivenoms and antitoxins
      8. Contrast media
      9. NSAIDs
   C. Neoplasms
      1. Hodgkin's disease
      2. Lymphoma
      3. Leukemia
      4. Carcinoma
      5. Melanoma
      6. Wilm's tumor

Continued

VI-17 DIFFERENTIAL DIAGNOSIS OF THE NEPHROTIC SYNDROME—*cont'd*

  D. Multisystem disease
- 1. Systemic lupus erythematosus
- 2. Henoch-Schönlein purpura
- 3. Vasculitis
- 4. Goodpasture's syndrome
- 5. Dermatomyositis
- 6. Dermatitis herpetiformis
- 7. Amyloidosis
- 8. Sarcoidosis
- 9. Sjögren's syndrome
- 10. Rheumatoid arthritis
- 11. Mixed connective tissue disease

  E. Heredofamilial
- 1. Diabetes mellitus
- 2. Alport's syndrome
- 3. Myxedema
- 4. Fabry's disease
- 5. Nail-patella syndrome
- 6. Lipodystrophy
- 7. Congenital nephrotic syndrome
- 8. Lecithin-cholesterol acyltransferase deficiency
- 9. Sickle cell disease

  F. Miscellaneous
- 1. Preeclamptic toxemia
- 2. Thyroiditis
- 3. Myxedema
- 4. Malignant obesity
- 5. Renovascular hypertension
- 6. Chronic interstitial nephritis with vesicoureteral reflux
- 7. Chronic allograft rejection
- 8. Bee stings

From Glassock R, Brenner R. In Isselbacher KJ et al (eds): *Harrison's principles of internal medicine,* ed 13, New York, 1994, McGraw-Hill, p. 1300.

VI-18 DIFFERENTIAL DIAGNOSIS OF TUBULOINTERSTITIAL DISEASE OF THE KIDNEY

I. Toxins
  A. Exogenous toxins
    1. Analgesic nephropathy
    2. Lead nephropathy
    3. Miscellaneous nephrotoxins (e.g., antibiotics, cyclosporine, radiographic contrast media, heavy metals)
  B. Metabolic toxins
    1. Acute uric acid nephropathy
    2. Gouty nephropathy
    3. Hypercalcemic nephropathy
    4. Hypokalemic nephropathy
    5. Miscellaneous metabolic toxins (e.g.,hyperoxaluria, cystinosis, Fabry's disease)
II. Neoplasia
  A. Lymphoma
  B. Leukemia
  C. Multiple myeloma
III. Immune disorders
  A. Hypersensitivity nephropathy
  B. Sjögren's syndrome
  C. Amyloidosis
  D. Transplant rejection
  E. Tubulointerstitial abnormalities associated with glomerulonephritis
  F. AIDS
IV. Vascular disorders
  A. Arteriolar nephrosclerosis
  B. Atheroembolic disease
  C. Sickle-cell nephropathy
  D. Acute tubular necrosis
V. Hereditary renal diseases
  A. Hereditary nephritis (Alport's syndrome)
  B. Medullary cystic disease
  C. Medullary sponge kidney
  D. Polycystic kidney disease
VI. Infectious injury
  A. Acute pyelonephritis
  B. Chronic pyelonephritis
VII. Miscellaneous disorders
  A. Chronic urinary tract obstruction
  B. Radiation nephritis
  C. Vesicoureteral reflux

From Brenner BM, Hosteter TH. In Isselbacher KJ et al (eds): *Harrison's principles of internal medicine,* ed 13, New York, 1994, McGraw-Hill, p. 1314.

VI-19   DIFFERENTIAL DIAGNOSIS OF NEPHROGENIC DIABETES INSIPIDUS

I. Congenital/familial
II. Renal disease
   A. Ureteral obstruction
   B. Polycystic disease
   C. Medullary cystic disease
   D. Pyelonephritis
   E. Advanced renal failure of any etiology
III. Electrolyte disorders
   A. Hypokalemia
   B. Hypercalcemia
IV. Drugs
   A. Alcohol
   B. Phenytoin
   C. Lithium
   D. Demeclocycline
   E. Acetohexamide
   F. Tolazamide
   G. Glyburide
   H. Propoxyphene
   I. Amphotericin
   J. Methoxyflurane
   K. Norepinephrine
   L. Vinblastine
   M. Cisplatin
   N. Colchicine
   O. Gentamicin
   P. Methicillin
   Q. Isophosphamide
   R. Contrast medium
   S. Osmotic diuretics
   T. Furosemide and ethacrynic acid
   U. Foscarnet
V. Systemic diseases
   A. Sickle cell disease
   B. Multiple myeloma
   C. Amyloidosis
   D. Sjögren's disease
   E. Sarcoidosis
VI. Dietary abnormalities
   A. Excessive water intake
   B. Decreased sodium chloride intake
   C. Decreased protein intake
VII. Pregnancy
VIII. Post urinary tract obstruction

From Berl T, Schrier RW. In Schrier RW (ed): *Renal and electrolyte disorders*, ed 4, Boston, 1992, Little, Brown, p. 37.

VI-20 DIFFERENTIAL DIAGNOSIS OF CENTRAL DIABETES INSIPIDUS

I. Idiopathic
  A. Sporadic
  B. Familial
II. Head trauma
III. Neurosurgical procedures
IV. Neoplasms
  A. Craniopharyngioma
  B. Meningitis
  C. Metastatic (e.g., breast cancer)
V. Lymphoma/leukemia
VI. Infection and granulomatous disease
  A. Encephalitis
  B. Meningitis
  C. Tuberculosis
  D. Syphilis
  E. Sarcoidosis
  F. Eosinophilic granuloma
VII. Vascular accidents
  A. Thrombosis
  B. Hemorrhage
  C. Sheehan's syndrome
VIII. Histiocytosis

From Oliver R, Jamison R: *Postgrad Medicine* 68:120, 1980.

VI-21   DIFFERENTIAL DIAGNOSIS OF HYPERURICEMIA

I. Overproduction of uric acid
   A. Primary gout
   B. Myeloproliferative disorders
   C. Lymphoma
   D. Hemoglobinopathies
   E. Hemolytic anemia
   F. Psoriasis
   G. Cancer chemotherapy
   H. Hypoxanthine phosphoribosyltransferase deficiency
   I. Phosphoribosylpyrophosphate synthetase deficiency
   J. Rhabdomyolysis
II. Underexcretion of uric acid
   A. Chronic renal failure
   B. Lead nephropathy (saturnine gout)
   C. Drugs
      1. Diuretics (except spironolactone)
      2. Ethambutol
      3. Aspirin
      4. Levodopa
      5. Pyrazinamide
      6. Nicotinic acid
      7. Cyclosporine
   D. Lactic acidosis (alcoholism, preeclampsia)
   E. Ketosis (diabetic, starvation)
   F. Hyperparathyroidism
   G. Hypertension
III. Overproduction and underexcretion of uric acid: Glycogen storage disease, Type I
IV. Mechanism unknown
   A. Sarcoidosis
   B. Obesity
   C. Hypoparathyroidism
   D. Paget's disease
   E. Down syndrome

From Beary JF, Scarpa NP: *Manual of rheumatology and outpatient orthopedics,* ed 2, Boston, 1987, Little, Brown, p. 153.

VI-22 DIFFERENTIAL DIAGNOSIS OF NEPHROLITHIASIS

I. Calcium stones
  A. Idiopathic hypercalciuria
  B. Hyperuricosuria
  C. Primary hyperparathyroidism
  D. Distal renal tubular acidosis (RTA)
  E. Hyperoxaluria
    1. Intestinal hyperoxaluria
    2. Hereditary
  F. Idiopathic stone disease
II. Uric acid stones
  A. Gout
  B. Idiopathic
  C. Dehydration
  D. Lesch-Nyhan syndrome
  E. Neoplasm
III. Cystine stones (hereditary)
IV. Struvite stones (infection)

From Coe F, Favus M. In Isselbacher KJ et al (eds): *Harrison's principles of internal medicine*, ed 13, New York, 1994, McGraw-Hill, p. 1330.

VI-23 DIFFERENTIAL DIAGNOSIS OF HYPOURICEMIA

I. Decreased production
  A. Congenital xanthine oxidase deficiency
  B. Liver disease
  C. Allopurinol administration
  D. Low PP-ribose-P synthetase activity
II. Increased excretion
  A. "Isolated" defect in renal transport of uric acid
    1. Idiopathic
    2. Neoplastic diseases
    3. Liver disease
  B. Generalized defect in renal tubular transport (Fanconi's syndrome)
    1. Idiopathic
    2. Wilson's disease
    3. Cystinosis
    4. Multiple myeloma
    5. Heavy metals
    6. Type I glycogen storage disease
    7. Galactosemia
    8. Hereditary fructose intolerance
    9. Outdated tetracyclines
    10. Bronchogenic carcinoma and other neoplasms
    11. Liver disease and alcoholism

Continued

VI-23 DIFFERENTIAL DIAGNOSIS OF HYPOURICEMIA—
cont'd

   C. Drugs
1. Acetoheximide
2. Azauridine
3. Benzbromarone
4. Benziodarone
5. Calcium ipodate
6. Chlorprothixene
7. Cinchophen
8. Citrate
9. Dicumarol
10. Diflumidone
11. Estrogens
12. Ethyl biscoumacetate
13. Ethyl p-chlorophenoxyisobutyric acid
14. Glyceryl guaiacolate
15. Glycine
16. Glycopyrrolate
17. Halofenate
18. Iodopyracet
19. Iopanoic acid
20. Meglumine iodipamide
21. p-Nitrophenylbutazone
22. Orotic acid
23. Outdated tetracycline
24. Phenolsulfonphthalein
25. Phenylbutazone
26. Phenylindanedione
27. Probenecid
28. Salicylates
29. Sodium diatrizoate
30. Sulfaethylthiadiazole
31. Sulfinpyrazone
32. W 2354
33. Zoxazolamine

  III. Mechanism unknown
    A. Pernicious anemia
    B. Acute intermittent porphyria

From Wyngaarden J, Kelley WM. In *Gout and urate metabolism,* New York, 1976, Grune & Stratton, p. 412.

VI-24   RENAL COMPLICATIONS OF NEOPLASMS

I. Glomerulonephritis, with or without nephrotic syndrome
II. Obstructive uropathy
    A. Tubular precipitation syndromes
        1. Uric acid nephropathy
        2. Hypercalcemic nephropathy
        3. Paraproteinuric syndromes
            a. Multiple myeloma
            b. Other (monoclonal gammopathy, lysozymuria, mucoproteins, proteolytic products)
    B. Obstruction of the ureters, bladder and urethra
III. Direct invasion by malignant process
    A. Primary renal tumors
    B. Metastatic infiltration
IV. Treatment-related nephropathies
    A. Radiation nephropathy
    B. Drug-induced nephrotoxicity
        1. Cytotoxic drugs
        2. Drugs used in supportive care
            a. Antibiotics
            b. Analgesics
        3. Immunotherapy
V. Miscellaneous
    A. Disseminated intravascular coagulation
    B. Amyloidosis
    C. Electrolyte abnormalities

From Fer et al: *Amer J Med* 71:705, 1981.

VI-25 CONDITIONS LEADING TO GENERALIZED EDEMA

   I. Kidney diseases
      A. Acute glomerulonephritis
      B. Nephrotic syndrome
      C. Acute renal failure
      D. Chronic renal failure
  II. Heart failure
 III. Liver diseases
      A. Cirrhosis
      B. Obstruction of hepatic venous outflow
  IV. Conditions confined to women
      A. Normal pregnancy
      B. Toxemia of pregnancy
      C. Idiopathic edema
   V. Vascular diseases
      A. Arteriovenous fistulas
      B. Obstruction of inferior or superior vena cava
  VI. Endocrine disorders
      A. Hypothyroidism
      B. Mineralocorticoid excess
      C. Diabetes mellitus
 VII. Iatrogenic disorders
      A. Drugs—oral contraceptives, estrogens, antihypertensives
      B. Excessive intravenous infusion of saline solutions
VIII. Miscellaneous
      A. Chronic hypokalemia
      B. Chronic anemia
      C. Nutritional edema
      D. Capillary leak syndrome
      E. Filariasis
      F. High-altitude edema

From Levy M, Seely JF. In Brenner B, Rector F: *The kidney*, ed 2, Philadelphia, 1981, WB Saunders, p. 726.

VI-26 CLINICAL SPECTRUM OF ABNORMALITIES IN UREMIA

I. Fluid and electrolyte disturbances
   A. Volume expansion and contraction
   B. Hypernatremia and hyponatremia
   C. Hyperkalemia and hypokalemia
   D. Metabolic acidosis
   E. Hyperphosphatemia and hypophosphatemia
   F. Hypocalcemia
II. Endocrine-metabolic disturbances
   A. Renal osteodystrophy
   B. Secondary hyperparathyroidism
   C. Carbohydrate intolerance
   D. Hyperuricemia
   E. Hypothermia
   F. Hypertriglyceridemia
   G. Protein-calorie malnutrition
   H. Impaired growth and development
   I. Infertility and sexual dysfunction
   J. Amenorrhea
   K. Osteomalacia
   L. Aluminum induced
   M. Vitamin D-deficient osteomalacia
   N. Dialysis (beta$_2$-microglobulin, amyloid) arthropathy
III. Neuromuscular disturbances
   A. Fatigue
   B. Sleep disorders
   C. Headache
   D. Impaired mentation
   E. Lethargy
   F. Asterixis
   G. Muscular irritability
   H. Peripheral neuropathy
   I. Restless leg syndrome
   J. Paralysis
   K. Myoclonus
   L. Seizures
   M. Coma
   N. Muscle cramps
   O. Dialysis disequilibrium syndrome
   P. Dialysis dementia
   Q. Myopathy

Continued

VI-26   CLINICAL SPECTRUM OF ABNORMALITIES
IN UREMIA—*cont'd*

IV. Cardiovascular and pulmonary disturbances
   A. Arterial hypertension
   B. Congestive heart failure or pulmonary edema
   C. Pericarditis
   D. Cardiomyopathy
   E. Uremic lung
   F. Accelerated atherosclerosis
   G. Hypotension and dysrhythmias
V. Dermatologic disturbances
   A. Pallor
   B. Hyperpigmentation
   C. Pruritus
   D. Ecchymoses
   E. Uremic frost
VI. Gastrointestinal disturbances
   A. Anorexia
   B. Nausea and vomiting
   C. Uremic fetor
   D. Gastroenteritis
   E. Peptic ulcer
   F. GI bleeding
   G. Hepatitis
   H. Refractory ascites on hemodialysis
   I. Peritonitis
VII. Hematologic and immunologic disturbances
   A. Normocytic, normochromic anemia
   B. Microcytic (aluminum-induced) anemia
   C. Lymphocytopenia
   D. Bleeding diathesis
   E. Increased susceptibility to infection
   F. Splenomegaly and hypersplenism
   G. Leukopenia
   H. Hypocomplementemia

From Brenner BM, Lazarus JM. In Isselbacher KJ et al (eds): *Harrison's principles of internal medicine*, ed 13, New York, 1994, McGraw-Hill, p. 1277.

VI-27 DIFFERENTIAL DIAGNOSIS OF RESPIRATORY ACIDOSIS

I. Acute respiratory acidosis
   A. Neuromuscular abnormalities
      1. Brain stem injury
      2. High cord injury
      3. Guillain-Barré
      4. Myasthenia gravis
      5. Botulism
      6. Narcotic, sedative or tranquilizer overdose
   B. Airway obstruction
      1. Foreign body
      2. Aspiration of vomitus
      3. Laryngeal edema
      4. Severe bronchospasm
   C. Thoracic-pulmonary disorders
      1. Flail chest
      2. Pneumothorax
      3. Severe pneumonia
      4. Smoke inhalation
      5. Severe pulmonary edema
   D. Massive pulmonary embolism
   E. Respirator controlled ventilation
      1. Inadequate frequency, tidal volume settings
      2. Large dead space
      3. Total parenteral nutrition
II. Chronic respiratory acidosis
   A. Neuromuscular abnormalities
      1. Chronic narcotic or sedative ingestion
      2. Primary hypoventilation
      3. Pickwickian syndrome
      4. Poliomyelitis
      5. Diaphragmatic paralysis
   B. Thoracic-pulmonary disorders
      1. Chronic obstructive airway disease
      2. Kyphoscoliosis
      3. End-stage interstitial pulmonary disease

From Kaehny WD. In Schrier RW (ed): Renal and electrolyte disorders, ed 4, Boston, 1992, Little, Brown, pp. 215-216.

VI-28   DIFFERENTIAL DIAGNOSIS OF RESPIRATORY ALKALOSIS

I. Central stimulation of respiration
   A. Anxiety
   B. Head trauma
   C. Brain tumors or vascular accidents
   D. Salicylates
   E. Fever
   F. Pain
   G. Pregnancy

II. Peripheral stimulation of respiration
   A. Pulmonary emboli
   B. Congestive heart failure
   C. Interstitial lung diseases
   D. Pneumonia
   E. "Stiff lungs" without hypoxemia
   F. Altitude
   G. Asthma

III. Uncertain
   A. Hepatic insufficiency
   B. Gram-negative septicemia

IV. Mechanical or voluntary hyperventilation

From Kaehny WG. In Schrier RW (ed): *Renal and electrolyte disorders*, ed 4, Boston, 1992, Little, Brown, p. 221.

VI-29   RULES OF THUMB FOR BEDSIDE INTERPRETATION OF ACID-BASE DISORDERS

Metabolic acidosis	$Paco_2$ should fall by 1.0 to 1.5 × the fall in plasma HCO_3 concentration
Metabolic alkalosis	$Paco_2$ should rise by 0.24 to 1.0 × the rise in plasma HCO_3 concentration
Acute respiratory acidosis	Plasma HCO_3 concentration should rise by about 1 mmol/L for each 10 mm Hg increment in $Paco_2$ (±3 mmol/L)
Chronic respiratory acidosis	Plasma HCO_3 concentration should rise about 4 mmol/L for each 10 mm Hg increment in $Paco_2$ (±4 mmol/L)
Acute respiratory alkalosis	Plasma HCO_3 concentration should fall by about 1 to 3 mmol/L for each 10 mm Hg decrement in the $Paco_2$, usually not to less than 18 mmol/L
Chronic respiratory alkalosis	Plasma HCO_3 concentration should fall by about 2 to 5 mmol/L per 10 mm Hg decrement in $Paco_2$ but usually not to less than 14 mmol/L

From Kaehny WG, Shapiro JI. In Schrier RW (ed): *Renal and electrolyte disorders*, ed 4, Boston, 1992, Little, Brown, p. 167.

VI-30   COMPLICATIONS OF DIALYSIS

Access	Dialysis procedure
Infection	Hemorrhage
Thrombosis	Hypotension
Vascular compromise	Cardiac ischemia
High-output CHF	Cramps, nausea, vomiting
Carpal tunnel syndrome	Seizures
Recirculation of blood flow	Hypoventilation, hypoxemia
	Anticoagulation
	Air embolism
	Hemolysis
	Dialysis disequilibrium syndrome
	Hypoglycemia

From Carpenter CB, Lazarus JM. In Wilson JD et al (eds): *Harrison's principles of internal medicine companion handbook,* ed 12, New York, 1991, McGraw-Hill, p. 388.

VI-31   CAUSES OF HEMATURIA

I. Glomerular causes of hematuria
  A. Proliferative diseases of the glomerulus
      1. Primary
          a. IgA nephropathy (Berger's disease)
          b. Poststreptococcal glomerulonephritis
          c. Membranoproliferative glomerulonephritis
          d. Idiopathic rapidly progressive glomerulonephritis
      2. Secondary (associated with multisystem diseases)
          a. Postinfectious glomerulonephritis
          b. Henoch-Schönlein purpura
          c. Systemic lupus erythematosus
          d. Goodpasture's syndrome
          e. Vasculitis
          f. Essential mixed cryoglobulinemia
  B. Nonproliferative diseases of the glomerulus
      1. Membranous glomerulopathy
      2. Focal and segmental glomerulosclerosis
      3. Diabetic glomerulosclerosis
  C. Familiar diseases of the glomerulus
      1. Alport's syndrome
      2. Thin basement membrane diseases
      3. Fabry's disease
      4. Nail-patella syndrome

Continued

VI-31   CAUSES OF HEMATURIA—*cont'd*

II. Nonglomerular renal parenchymal causes of hematuria
  A. Neoplasms
    1. Renal cell carcinoma
    2. Wilms' tumor
    3. Benign cysts
  B. Vascular
    1. Renal infarct
    2. Renal vein thrombosis
    3. Malignant hypertension
    4. Arteriovenous malformation
    5. Papillary necrosis
    6. Loin-pain hematuria syndrome
  C. Metabolic
    1. Hypercalciuria
    2. Hyperuricosuria
  D. Familial
    1. Polycystic kidney diseases
    2. Medullary sponge kidney
  E. Drugs
    1. Anticoagulants (heparin, warfarin)
    2. Drug-induced acute interstitial nephritis
  F. Trauma
  G. Papillary necrosis
    1. Analgesic abuse
    2. Sickle cell disease and trait
    3. Renal tuberculosis
    4. Diabetes
    5. Obstructive uropathy
III. Extrarenal causes of hematuria
  A. Calculi
    1. Ureter, bladder, prostate
  B. Neoplasms
    1. Transitional cell carcinoma (pelvis, ureter, and bladder)
    2. Adenocarcinoma and benign hypertrophy (prostate)
    3. Squamous cell carcinoma (urethra)
  C. Infections
    1. Acute cystitis, prostatitis, and urethritis
    2. Tuberculosis
    3. Schistosoma haematobium
  D. Drugs
    1. Anticoagulants (heparin, coumadin)
    2. Cyclophosphamide (hemorrhagic cystitis)
  E. Trauma

From Lieberthal W, Mesler DE. In Jacobson HR, Striker GE, Klahr S (eds): *The principles and practice of nephrology,* ed 2, St. Louis, 1995, Mosby, pp. 105-106.

VI-32   CAUSES OF RHABDOMYOLYSIS

I. Traumatic
   A. Crush injury
   B. Excessive muscle activity in sports
   C. Burns
   D. Ischemia
   E. Other
      1. Grand mal seizures
      2. Status asthmaticus
      3. Delirium tremens
      4. Military boot camp
II. Nontraumatic
   A. Toxins
      1. Ethanol
      2. Isopropyl alcohol
      3. Ethylene glycol
      4. Carbon monoxide
      5. Toluene
      6. Mercuric chloride
      7. Insect bite/sting
      8. Snake venom
   B. Metabolic disorders
      1. Diabetic ketoacidosis
      2. Nonketotic hyperosmolar coma
      3. Hypokalemia
      4. Hypernatremia
      5. Hypophosphatemia
      6. Hypomagnesemia
      7. Hypothermia
   C. Drugs
      1. Illicit (e.g., cocaine, heroin, LSD, amphetamines)
      2. Codeine
      3. Salicylate overdose
      4. Lovastatin
      5. Clofibrate
      6. Diphenhydramine
      7. Succinylcholine
      8. Barbiturate overdose
   D. Genetic disorders
      1. McArdle's syndrome (phosphorylase deficiency)
      2. Phosphofructokinase deficiency
      3. Phosphohexomerase deficiency
      4. Carnitine palmityl transferase deficiency
      5. Carnitine deficiency
      6. Muscular dystrophy

Continued

VI-32 CAUSES OF RHABDOMYOLYSIS—*cont'd*

E. Infectious diseases
1. Viral infections (Coxsackie, hepatitis, mononucleosis, influenza)
2. Tetanus
3. Gas gangrene
4. Legionnaire's disease
5. Shigellosis
6. Pseudomonas infection
7. Reye's syndrome

F. Other
1. Polymyositis
2. Dermatomyositis

From Bonventre JV, Shah SV, Walker PD, Hymphreys MH. In Jacobson HR, Striker GE, Klahr S (eds): *The principles and practice of nephrology,* ed 2, St. Louis, 1995, Mosby, p. 570.

VI-33 COMPLICATIONS OF ACUTE RENAL FAILURE

I. Metabolic
   A. Hyponatremia
   B. Hyperkalemia
   C. Hypocalcemia
   D. Hyperphosphatemia
   E. Hypermagnesemia
   F. Hyperuricemia

II. Cardiac
   A. Congestive heart failure or pulmonary edema
   B. Dysrhythmias
   C. Hypertension
   D. Pericarditis
   E. Myocardial infarction

III. Neurologic
   A. Asterixis
   B. Myoclonus
   C. Lethargy/somnolence
   D. Seizures
   E. Coma

IV. Hematologic
   A. Anemia
   B. Bleeding tendency
   C. Platelet dysfunction
   D. Leukocytosis

V. Gastrointestinal
   A. Nausea, vomiting, diarrhea
   B. Paralytic ileus
   C. GI bleed

VI. Infectious
   A. Pneumonia
   B. Urinary tract infection
   C. Wound infection
   D. Septicemia

VI-34 CLINICAL RISK FACTORS FOR CALCIUM STONE FORMATION

I. General issues and/or risk factors
   A. Positive family history
   B. Medications (vitamins A, D, C; absorbable antacids; acetazolamide)
   C. Urinary pH
   D. Diet
II. Specific, treatable risk factors
   A. Low urine volume
   B. Hypercalciuria
   C. Hyperoxaluria
   D. Hyperuricosuria
   E. Hypercitraturia

From Insogna KL, Broadus AE. In Felig P, Baxter JD, Broadus AE, Frohman LA (eds): *Endocrinology and metabolism,* ed 2, New York, 1987, McGraw-Hill, p 1529.

VI-35 CAUSES OF LACTIC ACIDOSIS

I. Decrease in tissue perfusion or oxygenation
   A. Septic shock
   B. Cardiogenic shock
   C. Hypovolemic shock
   D. Mesenteric vascular insufficiency
   E. Hypoxemia (respiratory failure)
   F. Large pulmonary emboli
   G. Severe anemia
II. Increased oxygen requirements
   A. Seizure
   B. Strenuous exercise (e.g., marathon running)
III. Systemic disorders
   A. Diabetes mellitus
   B. Liver failure
   C. Renal failure
   D. Malignancy (e.g., leukemia, lymphoma)
   E. Pregnancy
IV. Toxins
   A. Metformin
   B. Isoniazid
   C. Ethanol
   D. Methanol
   E. Ethylene glycol
   F. Carbon monoxide
   G. Cyanide
   H. Salicylates
   I. Iron overdose
V. Enzyme defects in glucose metabolism

CHAPTER VII

Pulmonary Disease

VII-1   DIFFERENTIAL DIAGNOSIS OF CLUBBING OF THE DIGITS

I. Pulmonary disorders
  A. Infection
    1. Bronchiectasis
    2. Lung abscess
    3. Empyema
    4. Tuberculosis (only with extensive fibrosis or abscess)
  B. Neoplasm
    1. Primary lung cancer
    2. Metastatic lung cancer
    3. Mesothelioma
    4. Hepatoma
  C. Pulmonary fibrosis
  D. Arteriovenous malformations
  E. Neurogenic diaphragmatic tumors
  F. Cystic fibrosis
II. Cardiac disorders
  A. Congenital cyanotic heart disease
  B. Infective endocarditis
III. Gastrointestinal disorders
  A. Ulcerative colitis
  B. Regional enteritis
  C. Hepatic cirrhosis
IV. Miscellaneous
  A. Hemiplegia

From Szidor JP, Fishman AP. In Fishman AP (ed): *Pulmonary diseases and disorders,* ed 2, vol 1, New York, 1988, McGraw-Hill, p. 318.

VII-2 DIFFERENTIAL DIAGNOSIS OF HEMOPTYSIS

I. Infections
  A. Bronchitis
  B. Bronchiectasis
  C. Pneumonia (especially Klebsiella)
  D. Lung abscess
  E. Tuberculosis
  F. Fungal
  G. Septic pulmonary emboli
II. Neoplasms
  A. Bronchogenic carcinoma
  B. Bronchial adenoma
III. Cardiovascular disorders
  A. Pulmonary infarction
  B. Mitral stenosis
  C. Pulmonary congestion and alveolar edema
  D. Aortic aneurysm
  E. Pulmonary arteriovenous fistula
  F. Primary pulmonary hypertension
  G. Eisenmenger's syndrome
IV. Trauma (including foreign body)
V. Miscellaneous
  A. Broncholithiasis
  B. Bleeding diathesis (including anticoagulant therapy)
  C. Goodpasture's syndrome
  D. Wegener's granulomatosis
  E. Cystic fibrosis

From Fishman AP. In Fishman AP (ed): *Pulmonary diseases and disorders,* ed 2, vol 1, New York, 1988, McGraw-Hill, p. 347.

VII-3 DIFFERENTIAL DIAGNOSIS OF BRONCHIECTASIS

I. Bronchopulmonary Infections
II. Bronchial obstruction
  A. Laryngeal papillomatosis
  B. Bronchogenic carcinoma
  C. Allergic bronchopulmonary aspergillosis
  D. Chronic bronchitis
III. Congenital/hereditary
  A. Williams-Campbell syndrome (cartilage deficiency)
  B. Mounier-Kuhn syndrome (tracheobronchomegaly)
  C. Pulmonary Sequestration
  D. Yellow-nail syndrome
  E. Immunodeficiency states
  F. Immotile cilia syndrome
  G. Kartagener's syndrome
  H. α_1-Antitrypsin deficiency
  I. Cystic fibrosis
IV. Miscellaneous
  A. Young's syndrome
  B. Recurrent aspiration

From Swartz M. In Fishman AP (ed): *Pulmonary diseases and disorders,* ed 2, vol 2, New York, 1988, McGraw-Hill, p. 1559.

VII-4 DIFFERENTIAL DIAGNOSIS OF PLEURAL EFFUSIONS*

I. Transudates
   A. Congestive heart failure
   B. Nephrotic syndrome
   C. Cirrhosis
   D. Peritoneal dialysis
   E. Meigs syndrome
   F. Hydronephrosis
   G. Myxedema
   H. Superior vena cava obstruction

II. Exudates
   A. Predominant
      1. Parapneumonic
      2. Malignancy
      3. Pulmonary embolization
   B. Common
      1. Tuberculosis
      2. Traumatic (including hemothorax)
      3. Pancreatitis
      4. Intraabdominal abscess
      5. Esophageal perforation
      6. After abdominal surgery
      7. Collagen vascular disease
         a. Rheumatoid arthritis
         b. Systemic lupus erythematosus
         c. Sjögren's syndrome
         d. Wegener's granulomatosis
   C. Unusual
      1. Drug-induced
         a. Nitrofurantoin
         b. Bromocriptine
         c. Amiodarone
      2. Asbestos
      3. Dressler's syndrome
      4. Fungal infection
      5. Chylothorax
      6. Uremia
      7. Radiation therapy
      8. Sarcoidosis
      9. Yellow-nail syndrome
      10. Trapped lung
      11. Ovarian hyperstimulation syndrome
      12. Mesothelioma

*Exudative pleural effusions must meet at least one of the following criteria:
1. Pleural fluid protein/serum protein >0.5.
2. Pleural fluid LDH/serum LDH >0.6.
3. Pleural fluid LDH >two thirds the upper limit for serum.

VII-5   CRITERIA FOR HOSPITALIZATION OF PATIENTS WITH PNEUMONIA

   I. Elderly (>65 years of age)
  II. Significant comorbidity (renal, heart, or lung disease; diabetes; neoplasm; immunosuppression)
 III. Leukopenia (<5,000 WBC per microliter)
 IV. Suspected pathogens: gram-negative bacilli, *Staphylococcus aureus,* or anaerobes
  V. Suppurative complications (empyema, arthritis, endocarditis)
 VI. Failure of outpatient management
 VII. Unable to tolerate oral intake
VIII. The following clinical signs:
     A. Tachypnea (>30 breaths/min)
     B. Hypotension
     C. Hypoxemia (PaO2 <60 mm Hg on room air)
     D. Altered mentation
     E. Bilateral lung involvement

From Philipson EA. In Isselbacher KJ et al (eds): *Harrison's principles of internal medicine,* ed 13, New York, 1994, McGraw-Hill, p. 1187.

VII-6   DIFFERENTIAL DIAGNOSIS OF COUGH WITH NEGATIVE CHEST X-RAY

  I. Acute respiratory infections
 II. Acute irritative bronchitis (inhaled or aspirated irritant)
    A. Exogenous irritants (tobacco smoke, smog, high levels of O_2, noxious gases in workplace)
    B. Mechanical irritants (foreign body, postnasal drip, gastric contents, retained bronchopulmonary secretions)
III. Postbronchitis cough syndrome
 IV. Chronic bronchitis
  V. Asthma
 VI. Bronchiectasis
VII. Congestive heart failure
VIII. Esophageal disease which results in recurrent aspiration
    A. Esophageal reflux
    B. Achalasia
    C. Zenker's diverticulum
 IX. Tracheobronchial neoplasms
    A. Primary tracheal neoplasms
    B. Secondary tracheal malignancy
    C. Bronchogenic carcinoma
    D. Bronchial adenoma
    E. Metastatic tumors
  X. Nonneoplastic bronchial obstructive lesions
    A. Foreign body
    B. Broncholithiasis
    C. Bronchial stricture
    D. Extrinsic compression
 XI. Cystic fibrosis
XII. Laryngeal lesions
XIII. Postnasal discharge
XIV. Psychogenic cough
XV. Pulmonary emboli

VII-7 DIFFERENTIAL DIAGNOSIS OF HILAR ENLARGEMENT

I. Unilateral
   A. Malignancy
      1. Primary bronchogenic carcinoma
      2. Metastatic lymphadenopathy
   B. Infections
      1. Tuberculosis
      2. Fungal
      3. Bacterial (occasionally)
   C. Sarcoidosis
   D. Lymph node hyperplasia
   E. Pulmonary artery enlargement
   F. Mediastinal masses
II. Bilateral
   A. Sarcoidosis
   B. Infection
      1. Tuberculosis
      2. Fungal
      3. Mononucleosis
      4. Mycoplasma
   C. Metastatic tumor
   D. Lymphoma
   E. Pneumoconioses
      1. Silicosis
      2. Berylliosis
   F. Vascular
      1. Enlargement of pulmonary arteries
         a. Pulmonary emboli
         b. Chronic cor pulmonale
      2. Enlargement of pulmonary veins
         a. Congestive heart failure
         b. Mitral stenosis

VII-8   DIFFERENTIAL DIAGNOSIS OF PNEUMOTHORAX

   I. Primary spontaneous pneumothorax
  II. Iatrogenic
 III. Traumatic
  IV. Mediastinal emphysema
   V. Pulmonary inflammation
      A. Tuberculosis
      B. Coccidioidomycosis (other fungal infections less commonly)
      C. Staphylococcal pneumonia with abscess (other bacterial pneumonias)
      D. *Pneumocystis carinii* pneumonia (PCP)
  VI. Rupture of cysts and bullae
 VII. "Honeycomb" lungs (pulmonary microcysts)
      A. Idiopathic
      B. Cystic fibrosis
      C. Scleroderma
      D. Eosinophilic granuloma
      E. Pulmonary tuberous sclerosis
      F. Pulmonary lymphangiomatoid granulomatosis
      G. Pneumoconioses
      H. Marfan's syndrome
VIII. Catamenial pneumothorax
  IX. Miscellaneous
      A. Asthma
      B. Pulmonary infarction with cavitation
      C. Eosinophilic
      D. Pseudoxanthoma elasticum
      E. Ehlers-Danlos
      F. Pulmonary hemosiderosis
      G. Paragonimiasis
      H. Pulmonary alveolar proteinosis
      I. Hydatid lung disease
      J. Rheumatoid lung disease

VII-9   DIFFERENTIAL DIAGNOSIS OF RECURRENT PULMONARY INFECTION ASSOCIATED WITH IMMUNODEFICIENCY SYNDROMES OTHER THAN HIV-RELATED

Immunodeficiency	Genetic	Acquired	Iatrogenic	Pulmonary pathogens
		Examples		
Humoral immunity	Common variable immunodeficiency Hypogammaglobulinemia	Multiple myeloma CLL	Cyclophosphamide Corticosteroids Irradiation	Encapsulated organism gram-negative bacilli
Phagocytosis	Chronic granulomatous disease	ALL Liver failure	Neutropenia secondary to drug therapy Hypersensitivity Rx	Bacteria and less-virulent organisms
				Aspergillus and other fungi
Cell-mediated immunity	DiGeorge's syndrome Severe combined Immunodeficiency Leucocyte activation	Systemic lupus erythematosus Lymphoma AIDS	Cytotoxic drugs Glucocorticoids Irradiation Cyclosporin Allogenic organ transplantation	Bacteria Fungi *P. Carini* Viruses HSV CMV EBV Legionella Nocardia

From Duncan SR, Raffin TA. In Murray JF, Nadel JA (eds): *Respiratory medicine*, ed 2, Philadelphia, 1995, WB Saunders, p. 2369.

VII-10 DIFFERENTIAL DIAGNOSIS OF EOSINOPHILIC LUNG DISEASE

I. Idiopathic
  A. Transient pulmonary eosinophilia (Loeffler's)
  B. Prolonged pulmonary eosinophilia (Carrington's)
II. Eosinophilic lung diseases of specific etiology
  A. Drug induced (i.e. nitrofurantoin and penicillin)
  B. Parasite induced
    1. Strongyloides
    2. Ancylostomiasis
    3. Tropical pulmonary eosinophilia
    4. Pulmonary larva migrans
    5. Schistosomiasis
    6. Toxocara
    7. Necator americanus
  C. Fungus induced
    1. Hypersensitivity bronchopulmonary aspergillosis
III. Eosinophilic lung disease associated with angiitis and/or granulomatosis
  A. Wegener's granulomatosis
  B. Allergic granulomatosis
  C. Polyarteritis nodosa
  D. Necrotizing alveolitis
  E. Necrotizing "sarcoidal" angiitis and granulomatosis

From Fraser RG, Para JA: *Diagnosis of diseases of the chest,* ed 3, vol 2, Philadelphia, 1988, WB Saunders, p. 1291.

VII-11 DIFFERENTIAL DIAGNOSIS OF PULMONARY INTERSTITIAL DISEASE

I. Occupational/environmental agents
  A. Inorganic dusts
    1. Silicosis
    2. Asbestosis
    3. Coal worker's pneumoconiosis
    4. Berylliosis
  B. Organic dusts
    1. Sugar cane
    2. Bird breeder's lung
    3. Farmer's lung
  C. Fumes
    1. Nitrogen dioxane
    2. Chlorine
    3. Ammonia
    4. Sulfur dioxide
II. Drugs
  A. Sulfonamides
  B. Bleomycin
  C. Busulfan
  D. Nitrofurantoin
  E. Gold salts
  F. Amiodarone
  G. Tocainide
  H. Penicillamine
  I. Methotrexate
  J. High-dose oxygen
  K. Crack cocaine inhalation
III. Radiation
IV. Infectious agents
  A. Viruses (influenza, CMV, varicella)
  B. Bacterial
  C. Fungal (histoplasmosis, coccidioidomycosis)
  D. Parasites (schistosomiasis, *Pneumocystis carinii*)
V. Cardiac disease (CHF)
VI. Metabolic abnormalities

From Jackson L, Fulmer J. In Fishman AP (ed): *Pulmonary diseases and disorders,* ed 2, vol 1, New York, 1988, McGraw-Hill, p. 740.

VII-12   DIFFERENTIAL DIAGNOSIS OF PULMONARY INTERSTITIAL DISEASE OF UNKNOWN ETIOLOGY

I. Connective tissue disease
   - A. Rheumatoid arthritis
   - B. Scleroderma
   - C. Sjögren's syndrome
   - D. Systemic lupus erythematosus
   - E. Polymyositis/dermatomyositis
   - F. Ankylosing spondylitis
   - G. Mixed connective tissue disease

II. Sarcoidosis

III. Amyloidosis

IV. Idiopathic fibrotis disorders
   - A. Idiopathic pulmonary fibrosis
   - B. Bronchiolitis obliterans organizing pneumonia
   - C. Autoimmune pulmonary fibrosis (inflammatory bowel disease, primary biliary cirrhosis)

V. Histiocytosis X

VI. Pulmonary hemorrhagic syndromes
   - A. Idiopathic hemosiderosis
   - B. Goodpasture's disease
   - C. Diffuse alveolar hemorrhage syndrome

VII. Malignancy
   - A. Lymphangitic carcinomatosis
   - B. Bronchoalveolar carcinoma
   - C. Pulmonary lymphoma.

VIII. Eosinophilic pneumonia/granuloma

IX. Alveolar proteinosis

X. Tuberous sclerosis

XI. Niemann-Pick disease

XII. Adult respiratory distress syndrome

XIII. Acquired immunodeficiency syndrome

XIV. Lymphangioleiomyomatosis

From Jackson L, Fulmer J. In Fishman AP (ed): *Pulmonary diseases and disorders,* ed 2, vol 1, New York, 1988, McGraw-Hill, p. 40.

VII-13 DIFFERENTIAL DIAGNOSIS OF RESPIRATORY FAILURE

I. Pulmonary origin
   A. Diffuse obstructive airway disease
   B. Central airway obstruction
   C. Restrictive lung disease
   D. Adult respiratory distress syndrome
   E. Pulmonary vascular disease
      1. Pulmonary embolus
      2. Arteriovenous fistula
      3. Venoocclusive disease
   F. Pleural and chest wall disease
      1. Pleural effusions
      2. Pleural fibrosis
      3. Pneumothorax
      4. Flail chest
      5. Fixed chest wall deformities
   G. Diaphragm muscle fatigue
   H. Metastatic tumor
   I. Infections
II. Extrapulmonary origin
   A. Neuromuscular disease
      1. Potentiated by electrolyte abnormalities ($\downarrow$K, $\downarrow$PO$_4$)
      2. Guillain-Barré
   B. Central nervous system disease
   C. Drug suppression of respiratory center
   D. Primary hypoventilation syndromes (sleep apnea syndromes)
      1. Central type
      2. Obstructive
      3. Mixed
   E. Laryngeal obstruction
   F. Congestive heart failure

VII-14 GUIDELINES FOR WITHDRAWAL OF MECHANICAL VENTILATION

I. An awake and alert mental state
II. PaO$_2$ >60 mm Hg, with FIO$_2$ $\leq$0.5
III. PEEP $\leq$5 cm H$_2$O
IV. PaCO$_2$ acceptable, with pH in the normal range
V. Vital capacity >10-15 mg/kg
VI. Minute ventilation <10 liters/min; respiratory rate <25/min
VII. Maximum voluntary ventilation double that of minute ventilation
VIII. Peak inspiratory pressure lower (more negative) than 25 cm H$_2$O
IX. Spontaneous ventilation via T tube (with or without CPAP) for 1 to 4 hours with acceptable blood gases and without marked increases in respiratory rate, heart rate, or change in general status

From Woodley M, Whelan A. In Orland MJ, Saltman RJ (eds): *Manual of medical therapeutics,* ed 27, Boston, 1992, Little, Brown, p. 191.

VII-15   DIFFERENTIAL DIAGNOSIS OF ALVEOLAR HYPERVENTILATION

I. Hypoxemia
   A. High altitude
   B. Pulmonary disease
II. Pulmonary disorders
   A. Pneumonia
   B. Interstitial pneumonitis, fibrosis, edema
   C. Pulmonary emboli
   D. Bronchial asthma
   E. Pneumothorax
III. Cardiovascular disorders
   A. Congestive heart failure
   B. Hypotension
IV. Metabolic disorders
   A. Acidosis (diabetic, renal, lactic)
   B. Hepatic failure
V. Neurologic disorders
   A. Psychogenic or anxiety hyperventilation
   B. CNS infection or tumor
VI. Drug-induced
   A. Salicylates
   B. Methylxanthine derivatives
   C. Beta-adrenergic agonists
   D. Progesterone
VII. Miscellaneous
   A. Fever, sepsis
   B. Pain
   C. Pregnancy

From Philipson EA. In Issselbacher, KJ et al (eds): *Harrison's principles of internal medicine,* ed 13, New York, 1994, McGraw-Hill, p. 1239.

VII-16 DIFFERENTIAL DIAGNOSIS OF CHRONIC ALVEOLAR HYPOVENTILATION

I. Functional depression of ventilatory drive
   A. Sleep
   B. Hypercapnia
   C. Metabolic alkalosis
   D. Prolonged hypoxia
   E. Drugs (narcotics, sedatives)
   F. Myxedema
   G. Carotid body dysfunction
II. Anatomic damage to respiratory neurons
   A. Bulbar poliomyelitis
   B. Encephalitis
   C. Brainstem infarction
   D. Brainstem neoplasm
   E. Brainstem demyelination
   F. Bilateral cervical cordotomy
III. Idiopathic alveolar hypoventilation
IV. Organic depression of motor pathways (Ondine's curse)
V. Peripheral neuromuscular disorders
   A. Poliomyelitis
   B. Guillain-Barré syndrome
   C. Myasthenia gravis
   D. Muscular dystrophy
   E. Polymyositis
   F. Bilateral diaphragmatic paralysis
VI. Disorders of the chest cage
   A. Kyphoscoliosis
   B. Obesity-hypoventilation syndromes
   C. Thoracoplasty
   D. Anchylosing spondylitis
VII. Obstruction of the upper airways
   A. Tracheal stenosis
   B. Obstructive sleep apnea
   C. Cystic fibrosis
   D. Chronic obstructive pulmonary disease

VII-17   SYMPTOMS AND SIGNS OBSERVED IN 327 PATIENTS WITH ANGIOGRAPHICALLY DOCUMENTED PULMONARY EMBOLI

Symptoms and signs	%
Symptoms	
Chest pain	88
Pleuritic	74
Nonpleuritic	14
Dyspnea	85
Apprehension	59
Cough	53
Hemoptysis	30
Sweats	27
Syncope	13
Signs	
Respirations >16/min.	92
Rales	58
Increased S_2P*	53
Pulse >100 min.	44
Temperature >37.8°C	43
Diaphoresis	36
Gallop	34
Phlebitis	32
Edema	24
Murmur	23
Cyanosis	19

*Increased S_2P = increase in intensity of the pulmonic component of the second heart sound.
From Bell WR, Simon TS, DeMets DL: *Am J Med* 62:355, 1977.

VII-18 ECG CHANGES IN PULMONARY EMBOLISM

ECG changes	Percentage
Normal sinus rhythm or sinus tachycardia	75% to 80%
Rhythm changes	20% to 25%
Premature atrial contractions	10%
Premature ventricular contractions	10%
Atrial fibrillation	5%
Conduction disturbance	10%
QRS axis changes	
Acute right shift (S_1Q_3 pattern)	15%
Right bundle branch block	8%
T changes	40%
Depressed ST segments	25%
Elevated ST segments	16%

From Stein PD et al: *Progr Cardiovasc Dis* 17:247, 1974.

VII-19   CLINICAL DISORDERS ASSOCIATED WITH THE ADULT RESPIRATORY DISTRESS SYNDROME

I. Sepsis
II. Trauma
   A. Fat emboli
   B. Lung contusion
   C. Massive blood transfusions
III. Liquid aspiration
   A. Gastric contents
   B. Fresh and salt water (drowning)
   C. Hydrocarbon fluids
IV. Drug-associated
   A. Heroin
   B. Cocaine
   C. Ethchlorvynol
   D. Aspirin
V. Inhaled toxins
   A. Smoke
   B. Corrosive chemicals (NO_2, CL_2, NH_3, phosgene)
VI. Shock of any etiology
VII. Hematologic disorders
   A. Thrombocytopenic purpura
   B. Disseminated intravascular coagulation
VIII. Metabolic
   A. Acute pancreatitis
IX. Miscellaneous
   A. Lymphangiography
   B. Reexpansion pulmonary edema
   C. Neurogenic pulmonary edema
   D. Postcardiopulmonary bypass
   E. Eclampsia
   F. Air emboli
   G. Amniotic fluid embolism
   H. Ascent to high altitude

From Matthay MA: *Clin Chest Med* 6:311, 1985.

VII-20 PROGNOSTIC INDICATORS IN PNEUMOCOCCAL PNEUMONIA

I. Multilobe involvement (hypoxia)
II. Metastatic sites of infection, such as bone, pericardium, meningitis (positive blood cultures)
III. Immunocompromised states
    A. Hodgkin's and non-Hodgkin's lymphoma
    B. Leukemia
    C. Corticosteroid use
IV. Asplenic states (sickle cell anemia, postsplenectomy)
V. HIV infection
VI. WBC <5000 or >25,000
VII. Extremes of age (<1 year and >55 years)
VIII. Complement abnormalities
IX. Agammaglobulinemia
X. Preexisting illnesses (chronic lung disease, diabetes mellitus)
XI. Ethanolism
XII. Pneumococci demonstrated on peripheral smear

VII-21 CLASSIFICATION OF LUNG ABSCESSES ACCORDING TO CAUSE

I. Necrotizing infections
    A. Pyogenic bacteria (*Stapylococcus aureus*, Klebsiella, group A streptococcus, Bacteroides, Fusobacterium, anaerobic and microaerophilic cocci and streptococci, other anaerobes, Nocardia)
    B. Mycobacteria *(Mycobacterium tuberculosis, M. kansasii, Pseudomonas aeruginosa*, Legionella, *M. avium-intracellulare)*
    C. Fungi (Histoplasma, Coccidioides, Aspergillus)
    D. Parasites (amoeba, lung flukes)
II. Cavitary infarction
    A. Bland embolism
    B. Septic embolism (various anaerobes, Staphylococcus, Candida)
    C. Vasculitis (Wegener's granulomatosis, polyarteritis)
III. Cavitary malignancy
    A. Primary bronchogenic carcinoma
    B. Metastatic malignancies (very uncommon)
IV. Other
    A. Infected cysts
    B. Necrotic conglomerate lesions (silicosis, coal miner's pneumoconiosis)

From Reynolds H. In Wilson JD et al (eds): *Harrison's principles of internal medicine,* ed 12, New York, 1991, McGraw-Hill, p. 1068.

VII-22   CRITERIA FOR THE DIAGNOSIS OF ALLERGIC BRONCHOPULMONARY ASPERGILLOSIS

I. Primary
  A. Asthma
  B. Peripheral blood and sputum eosinophilia
  C. Positive immediate skin test
  D. Positive serum precipitins
  E. Elevated IgE levels
  F. Recurrent pulmonary infiltrates
  G. Central bronchiectasis on bronchograms
II. Secondary
  A. Aspergillus in sputum on repeated culture
  B. Expectoration of "brown plugs"
  C. Positive 6 to 8 hour delayed skin test

Note: The first six primary signs should be present for the diagnosis to be made.

From Corrigan K, Kory R: *Ann Intern Med* 86:405, 1977.

VII-23   SOLITARY PULMONARY NODULES

I. Differential diagnosis of a solitary pulmonary nodule*
  A. Malignant neoplasm
    1. Primary lung carcinoma or sarcoma
    2. Metastatic carcinoma or sarcoma
  B. Inflammation
    1. Granulomas
    2. Inflammatory pseudotumor
    3. Localized scar
  C. Benign neoplasms
    1. "Hamartoma"
    2. Other mesenchymal tumors
    3. Clear cell ("sugar") tumor
  D. Malformation
    1. Pulmonary sequestration
II. Common nonmalignant lesions presenting as solitary pulmonary nodules†
  A. Very common
    1. Granulomas
       a. Histoplasmoma, tuberculoma, coccidioidoma
       b. Cryptococcosis, blastomycosis, actinomycosis
    2. Unidentified granulomas
  B. Common
    1. Lung abscess before evacuation into a bronchus
    2. Slowly resolving circumscribed pneumonia
    3. Lipoid pneumonia
    4. Hamartoma
  C. Less common
    1. Bronchogenic cyst
    2. Pulmonary infarct
    3. Bronchial adenoma
    4. A-V fistula
    5. Enlarged pulmonary artery
    6. Infected, fluid-filled bulla
    7. Rheumatoid nodule

*From Oches RN. In Fishman AP (ed): *Pulmonary diseases and disorders,* ed 2, vol 3, New York, 1988, McGraw-Hill, p. 2019.
†From Rohwedder JJ. In Guenter CA, Welch MH (eds): *Pulmonary medicine,* ed 2, Philadelphia, 1982, JB Lippincott, p. 843.

VII-24 DIFFERENTIAL DIAGNOSIS OF TUMORS METASTATIC TO THE LUNGS

I. Parenchymal nodules
  A. Solitary carcinoma
    1. Large bowel
    2. Breast
    3. Kidney
    4. Female genital tract
    5. Skin
  B. Solitary sarcoma
    1. Osteogenic
  C. Multiple nodules
    1. Any carcinoma
    2. Any sarcoma
II. Endobronchial metastases
  A. Carcinoma
    1. Kidney
    2. Large bowel
  B. Fibrosarcoma
  C. Malignant melanoma
III. Lymphangitic metastases (carcinomas)
  A. Lung
  B. Stomach
  C. Breast
  D. Large bowel
  E. Pancreas

From Ochs R. In Fishman AP (ed): *Pulmonary diseases and disorders,* ed 2, vol 3, New York, 1988, McGraw-Hill, p. 2022.

VII-25 DIFFERENTIAL DIAGNOSIS OF A MEDIASTINAL MASS

I. Situated predominantly in the anterior compartment
   A. Thymoma
   B. Germ cell neoplasm
      1. Teratoma
      2. Seminoma
      3. Primary choriocarcinoma
      4. Endodermal sinus tumor
   C. Thyroid masses
   D. Parathyroid masses
   E. Mesenchymal neoplasms
      1. Lipoma
      2. Fibroma
      3. Hemangioma
      4. Lymphangioma
      5. Angiosarcoma
II. Situated predominantly in the middle compartment
   A. Lymph node enlargement caused by lymphoma or leukemia
   B. Lymph node enlargement caused by metastatic carcinoma
   C. Lymph node enlargement caused by infections
      1. Fungal
      2. Tuberculosis
      3. Mononucleosis
   D. Lymph node enlargement caused by granulomatous disease
   E. Primary tracheal neoplasms
   F. Bronchogenic cyst
   G. Masses situated in the anterior cardiophrenic angle
   H. Dilatation of the main pulmonary artery
   I. Dilatation of the major mediastinal veins
   J. Dilatation of the aorta or its branches
III. Situated predominantly in the posterior compartment
   A. Neurogenic neoplasms
   B. Meningocele
   C. Neurenteric cysts
   D. Gastroenteric cysts
   E. Thoracic duct cysts
   F. Primary lesions of the esophagus
      1. Neoplasm
      2. Diverticula
      3. Megaesophagus
      4. Hiatal hernia
   G. Hernia through the foramen of Bochdalek
   H. Diseases of the thoracic spine
      1. Neoplasms
      2. Infectious spondylitis
      3. Fracture with hematoma
   I. Extramedullary hematopoiesis

From Fraser RG, Para JA. In Fraser RG et al (eds): *Diagnosis of diseases of the chest,* ed 3, vol IV, Philadelphia, 1991, WB Saunders, p. 2794.

VII-26   PULMONARY MANIFESTATIONS OF THE COLLAGEN-VASCULAR DISEASES

Pulmonary manifestations	Rheumatoid arthritis	Systemic sclerosis	Polymyositis and dermatomyositis	Systemic lupus erythematosus	Mixed connective tissue disease
Pleural					
Thickening	++	+	0	++	0
Effusion	++	0	0	+++	0
Parenchymal					
Acute pneumonia	0	0	0	+	0
Interstitial fibrosis	++*	+++	++*	+	++
Nodules	++	0	0	0	0
Primary pulm vasculopathy	0	++	0	+	+
Aspiration	0	++	+++	0	0
Ventilatory insufficiency	0	+	++	+	0

*A rapidly progressing variant may occur.

NOTE: O = Absent or rare; + = uncommon; ++ = recognized manifestation; +++ = important feature of disease.

From Dickey B, Myers A. In Fishman AP (ed): *Pulmonary diseases and disorders*, ed 2, vol 1 New York, 1988, McGraw-Hill, p. 646.

VII-27   PULMONARY-RENAL SYNDROMES

I. Goodpasture's syndrome (antiglomerular membrane disease)
II. Vasculitides
III. Polyarteritis nodosa
IV. Churg-Strauss
V. Hypersensitivity angiitis (Zeek's syndrome, Henoch-Schönlein purpura, essential mixed cryoglobulinemia, "collagen diseases," malignancy, liver disease)
VI. Wegener's granulomatosis
VII. Lymphomatoid granulomatosis
VIII. Behçet's syndrome
IX. Systemic lupus erythematosus
X. Progressive systemic sclerosis (scleroderma)
XI. Mixed connective tissue disease

From Matthay RA: *Yale J Biol Med* 53:497, 1980.

VII-28   IMITATORS OF PULMONARY-RENAL SYNDROMES

I. Infections
   A. Bacterial endocarditis with pneumonitis and GN
   B. Streptococcal pneumonia with GN
   C. Staphylococcal pneumonia/abscess with GN
   D. Tuberculosis
   E. Leprosy
   F. Leptospirosis
   G. Legionnaires
   H. Hepatitis B
II. Sarcoidosis
III. CHF
IV. ARDS and ARF
V. Drugs
VI. Renal vein thrombosis with pulmonary embolism
VII. Plasma cell dyscrasia
VIII. Amyloid
IX. Fabry's disease

From Matthay RA: *Yale J Biol Med* 53:497, 1980.

VII-29 DIFFERENTIAL DIAGNOSIS OF FEVER AND PULMONARY INFILTRATES IN RENAL TRANSPLANTS*

CXR	Acute (<24 hrs)	Chronic (days-weeks)
Focal/multifocal	Bacterial	Fungal
	Thromboembolic	Nocardial
	Pulmonary edema	TB
Diffuse	Pulmonary edema	Viral
		Pneumocystis
Nodular	(Bacterial, pulmonary edema)	(Fungal)
		Nocardial
Peribronchovascular	Pulmonary edema	Viral
	(Bacterial)	Pneumocystis
Consolidation	Bacterial	Fungal
	Thromboembolic	Nocardial
	(Pulmonary edema)	(Viral)

(. . .) represents atypical manifestations.
*Pulmonary embolic disease and edema account for 27%.
*96% mortality for patients developing a secondary infection
From Roasey PG et al: *Medicine* 59:206, 1980.

VII-30   DRUGS IMPLICATED IN THE ETIOLOGY OF PULMONARY PARENCHYMAL INJURY

Cytotoxic	Noncytotoxic
I. Antibiotics	I. Antibacterial
A. Bleomycin	A. Nitrofurantoin
B. Mitomycin	B. Amphotericin
C. Neocarzinostatin	C. Sulfasalazine
II. Alkylating agents	II. Analgesics
A. Busulfan	A. Aspirin
B. Cyclophosphamide	III. Opiates
C. Chlorambucil	A. Heroin
D. Melphalan	B. Propoxyphene
III. Nitrosoureas	C. Methadone
A. Carmustine (BCR/U)	IV. Sedatives
B. Lomostine (CCR/U)	A. Ethchlorvynol
C. Chlorozotocin	B. Chlordiazepoxide
	V. Anticonvulsants
IV. Antimetabolites	A. Diphenylhydantoin
A. Methotrexate	B. Carbamazepine
B. Azathioprine	VI. Diuretics
C. Mercaptopurine	A. Hydrochlorothiazide
D. Cytosine arabinoside	VII. Major Tranquilizers
V. Miscellaneous	A. Haloperidol
A. Procarbazine	B. Fluphenazine
B. Vinblastine	VIII. Antiarrhythmics
	A. Amiodarone
	B. Lidocaine
	C. Tocainide
	IX. Miscellaneous
	A. Gold salts
	B. Penicillamine
	C. Colchicine
	D. Redux

From Cooper JAD et al: *Am Rev Respir Dis* 133:322; 1986.

VII-31 MULTI-ORGAN SYSTEM FAILURE*: MODIFIED APACHE II CRITERIA

I. Cardiovascular failure
   A. Heart rate $\leq$54/min
   B. Mean arterial blood pressure <49 mm Hg (systolic blood pressure $\leq$60 mm Hg)
   C. Ventricular tachycardia and/or fibrillation
   D. Serum pH $\leq$7.24 with pCO_2 of $\leq$49 mm Hg

II. Respiratory failure
   A. Respiratory rate $\leq$5/min or $\geq$49/min
   B. pCO_2 $\geq$50 mm Hg
   C. $AaDO_2$ $\geq$350 mm Hg
      ($AaDO_2$ = 713 FIO_2 − pCO_2 − pO_2)
   D. Ventilator or CPAP dependent 48 hours after appearance of another criterion

III. Renal failure†
   A. Urine output $\leq$479 ml/24 hours or $\leq$159 ml/8 hours
   B. Serum BUN $\geq$100 mg/100 ml
   C. Serum creatinine $\geq$3.5 mg/100 ml

IV. Hematologic failure
   A. WBC $\leq$1,000 cu mm
   B. Platelets $\leq$20,000 cu mm
   C. Hematocrit $\leq$20%

V. Neurologic failure
   A. Glasgow Coma Score $\leq$6 (in absence of sedation)

VI. Liver failure
   A. Bilirubin >6 mg%
   B. PT >4 sec over control

*Presence of any one or more of the criteria during a 24-hour period signifies organ failure.
†Excluding patients on chronic dialysis before hospitalization.
From Knaus WA, Wagner DP: *Crit Care Clin* 5(2):223, April 1989.

CHAPTER VIII

Clinical Immunology and Rheumatology

VIII-1   DIAGNOSTIC CRITERIA FOR SYSTEMIC LUPUS ERYTHEMATOSUS*

   I. Malar rash
  II. Discoid rash
 III. Photosensitivity
  IV. Oral or nasopharyngeal ulcers
   V. Arthritis
  VI. Serositis
       A. Pleuritis *or*
       B. Pericarditis
 VII. Renal disorder
       A. Proteinuria >0.5 grams/day *or*
       B. Cellular cases
VIII. Neurologic disorder
       A. Seizures *or*
       B. Psychosis
  IX. Hematologic disorder, one of the following:
       A. Hemolytic anemia
       B. Leukopenia
       C. Lymphopenia
       D. Thrombocytopenia
   X. Immunologic disorder, one of the following:
       A. Positive LE prep
       B. Antibody to DNA
       C. Antibody to SM
       D. False positive serologic test for syphilis
  XI. Antinuclear antibody in abnormal titer

*Four or more are required for the diagnosis of systemic lupus erythematosus.

From Tan EM et al: *Arthritis Rheum* 25:1271-1277, 1982.

VIII-2 UNDERLYING CONDITIONS ASSOCIATED WITH RAYNAUD'S PHENOMENON

I. Connective tissue diseases
   A. Scleroderma
   B. Lupus erythematosus
   C. Dermatomyositis
   D. Rheumatoid arthritis
   E. Mixed connective tissue disease
   F. Sjögren's syndrome
II. Neurogenic disorders
   A. Thoracic outlet syndrome
   B. Carpal tunnel syndrome
   C. Reflex sympathetic dystrophy
III. Vasoocclusive disease
   A. Arteriosclerosis obliterans
   B. Thromboangiitis obliterans
   C. Peripheral emboli
IV. Hematologic disorders
   A. Cryoglobulinemia
   B. Cold agglutinins
   C. Dysproteinemias
V. Drugs
   A. Ergot
   B. Heavy metal intoxications (lead and arsenic)
   C. Propranolol
   D. Sulfasalazine
VI. Occupational or environmental exposure
   A. Pneumatic hammer disease
   B. Disorders in typists and pianists
   C. Sequelae of blunt trauma or cold injury
VII. Miscellaneous
   A. Polycythemia vera
   B. Hypothyroidism
   C. Occult carcinoma
   D. Primary pulmonary hypertension
   E. Primary/idiopathic

From Creager MA, Dzau VJ. In Isselbacher KJ et al (eds): *Harrison's principles of internal medicine*, ed 13, New York, 1994, McGraw-Hill, p. 1994.

VIII-3   POLYMYALGIA RHEUMATICA

I. Diagnostic Criteria
- A. Musculoskeletal pain in neck, shoulders, and pelvic girdle for at least 1 month
- B. Patients usually at least 60 years of age
- C. Elevated ESR (usually greater than 50)
- D. Frequently present:
  - 1. Anemia
  - 2. Headache
  - 3. Morning stiffness >1 hour
  - 4. Depression and/or weight loss

II. Differential diagnosis
- A. Connective tissue disorders
  - 1. Rheumatoid arthritis
  - 2. Polymyositis
  - 3. Vasculitis
  - 4. Lupus erythematosus
- B. Neoplastic disorders
  - 1. Multiple myeloma
  - 2. Occult tumors
- C. Infections
  - 1. Post viral syndromes (especially, influenza)
  - 2. Occult infection
- D. Miscellaneous
  - 1. Degenerative joint disease
  - 2. Fibromyalgia

VIII-4   CRITERIA FOR DIAGNOSIS OF STEVENS-JOHNSON SYNDROME

I. Major criteria
- A. Skin lesions
- B. Erythema multiforme exudativum
- C. Stomatitis (ulcerative)
- D. Genital or anal ulcers

II. Minor criteria
- A. Pneumonitis—preceding or coexistent
- B. History of upper respiratory or genitourinary infection treated with sulfonamides or antibiotics
- C. Arthralgias
- D. Conjunctivitis
- E. History of ingestion of wide variety of drugs, both prescription and nonprescripton

From Ehrlich G. In McCarty DJ (ed): *Arthritis and allied conditions,* Philadelphia, 1985, Lea & Febiger, p. 896.

VIII-5 DIAGNOSTIC CRITERIA FOR BEHÇET'S SYNDROME*

I. Oral ulcerations (recurrent aphthous ≥3 attacks/year) PLUS ANY *TWO* OF THE FOLLOWING:
   A. Genital ulceration (recurrent aphthous)
   B. Eye inflammation
      1. Uveitis
         a. Anterior
         b. Posterior
      2. Vitreous cells on slit lamp
      3. Retinal vasculitis
   C. Skin lesions
      1. Erythema nodosum
      2. Pseudo-folliculitis
      3. Papulo-pustular
      4. Acneiform nodules
   D. Pathergy test (2 mm erythema 24 to 48 hours after no. 25 needle pricked to depth of 5 mm)

*For inclusion, each criterion must be confirmed by a physician.

From Duffy JD. In Schumacher HR, Klippel JH, Koopman WJ (eds): *Primer on the rheumatic diseases,* ed. 10, Atlanta, 1993, Arthritis Foundation, p. 206.

VIII-6 CRITERIA FOR THE DIAGNOSIS OF SCLERODERMA (Progressive Systemic Sclerosis)

I. Single major criterion—proximal scleroderma*
II. Minor criteria
   A. Sclerodactyly
   B. Digital pitting of finger tips
   C. Bibasilar pulmonary fibrosis

*Term indicating bilateral and symmetric sclerodermatous changes in any area proximal to the metacarpal or metatarsal phalangeal joints. The diagnosis of definite scleroderma can be made with one major or two or more minor criteria.

From Masi AT et al: *Arthritis Rheum* 23:581, 1980.

VIII-7   DIAGNOSTIC CRITERIA FOR INFLAMMATORY MYOPATHIES

Criterion	Polymyositis		Dermatomyositis		Inclusion-body myositis Definite
	Definite	Probable*	Definite	Mild or early	
Muscle strength	Myopathic muscle weakness†	Myopathic muscle weakness†	Myopathic muscle weakness†	Seemingly normal strength‡ of distal muscles†	Myopathic muscle weakness with early involvement
Electromyographic findings	Myopathic	Myopathic	Myopathic or nonspecific	Myopathic potentials	Myopathic with mixed
Muscle enzymes	Elevated (up to 50-fold)	Elevated (up to 50-fold) or normal	Elevated (up to 50-fold) or normal	Elevated (up to 10-fold) or normal	Elevated (up to 10-fold) or normal
Muscle biopsy findings	Diagnostic for this type of inflammatory myopathy	Nonspecific myopathy without signs of primary inflammation	Diagnostic	Nonspecific or diagnostic	Diagnostic
Rash or calcinosis	Absent	Absent	Present	Present	Absent

*An adequate trial of prednisone or other immunosuppressive drugs is warranted in probable cases. If, in retrospect, the disease is unresponsive to therapy, another muscle biopsy should be considered to exclude other diseases or possible evolution to inclusion body myositis.
†Myopathic muscle weakness, affecting proximal muscles more than distal ones and sparing eye and facial muscles, is characterized by a subacute onset (weeks to months) and rapid progression in patients who have no family history of neuromuscular disease, no endocrinopathy, no exposure to myotoxic drugs or toxins, and no biochemical muscle disease (excluded on the basis of muscle-biopsy findings).
‡Although strength is seemingly normal, patients often have new onset of easy fatigue, myalgia, and reduced endurance. Careful muscle testing may reveal mild muscle weakness.
From Dalakas MC: *New Engl J Med* 325(21):1490, 1991.

VIII-8 REVISED CRITERIA FOR CLASSIFICATION OF RHEUMATOID ARTHRITIS (TRADITIONAL FORMAT)*

Criterion	Definition
Morning stiffness	Morning stiffness in and around the joints, lasting at least 1 hour before maximal improvement.
Arthritis of 3 or more joint areas	At least 3 joint areas simultaneously have had soft tissue swelling or fluid (not bony overgrowth alone) observed by a physician. The 14 possible areas are right or left PIP, MCP, wrist, elbow, knee, ankle, and MTP joints.
Arthritis of hand joints	At least 1 area swollen (as defined above) in a wrist, MCP, or PIP joint.
Symmetric arthritis	Simultaneous involvement of the same joint areas (as defined in 2) on both sides of the body.
Rheumatoid nodules	Subcutaneous nodules, over bony prominences, or extensor surfaces, or in juxtaarticular regions, observed by a physician.
Serum rheumatoid factor	Demonstration of abnormal amounts of serum rheumatoid factor by any method for which the result has been positive in <5% of normal control subjects
Radiographic changes	Radiographic changes typical of rheumatoid arthritis on posteroanterior hand and wrist radiographs, which must include erosions or unequivocal bony decalcification localized in or most markedly adjacent to the involved joints (osteoarthritis changes alone do not qualify)

*For classification purposes, a patient shall be said to have rheumatoid arthritis if he/she has satisfied at least 4 of these 7 criteria. Criteria 1 through 4 must have been present for at least 6 weeks. Patients with 2 clinical diagnoses are not excluded. Designation as classic, definite, or probable rheumatoid arthritis is *not* to be made.

PIP, Proximal interphalangeal; *MCP,* metacarpophalangeal; *MTP,* metatarsophalangeal.

From Arnett FC, Edworthy SM, Bloch DA, et al: *Arthritis Rheum* 31: 315-324, March 1988.

VIII-9   CLINICAL FEATURES SUGGESTING REITER'S SYNDROME

I. History of diarrhea or extramarital sexual intercourse prior to attack
II. Fever
III. Arthritis, usually pauciarticular
IV. Urethritis, possibly complicated by cystitis, prostatic abscess or hydronephrosis
V. Conjunctivitis, possibly complicated by keratitis, iritis, retinitis or optic neuritis
VI. Skin lesions
   A. Keratoderma blennorhagicum
   B. Circinate balanitis
   C. Superficial ulcerations on tongue and buccal mucosa
VII. Possible ECG changes, infrequently pericarditis

From Yu DT, Hoffman RW. In Schumacher HR Jr (ed): *Primer on the rheumatic diseases*, ed 9, Atlanta, 1988, Arthritis Foundation, pp. 147-148.

VIII-10   DIAGNOSTIC CRITERIA OF ANKYLOSING SPONDYLITIS*

I. Clinical criteria
   A. Low back pain of over 3 months' duration, unrelieved by rest, improved with exercise
   B. Limited chest expansion
   C. Limited motion of the lumbar spine
   D. Past or present evidence of iritis.
II. Radiologic criteria
   A. Bilateral sacroiliitis grade 2-4
   B. Unilateral sacroiliitis grade 3-4

*Definite ankylosing spondylitis if either radiologic criterion present with one clinical criterion.

From Felson DT. In McCarty DJ (ed): *Arthritis and allied conditions*, ed 12, Philadelphia, 1993, Lea & Febiger, p. 26.

VIII-11 CRITERIA FOR DIAGNOSIS OF GOUTY ARTHRITIS

I. Patient with six or more of the following variable positives would be classified as having gout:
   A. Monoarticular arthritis
   B. Occurrence of more than one attack
   C. Maximal inflammation developing within one day
   D. Redness over joints
   E. Pain or swelling in the first metatarsophalangeal joint
   F. Unilateral involvement of E above
   G. Unilateral involvement of a tarsal joint
   H. Tophus—either proved or suspected to contain MSU crystals
   I. Serum uric acid >normal for that particular lab
   J. X-ray demonstrated asymmetric joint swelling
   K. Subcortical cysts without erosions on x-ray
   L. Monosodium urate crystals in joint fluid
   M. Joint fluid negative for organisms

II. Synovial fluid MSU crystals of proved tophus are universally accepted as the ultimate diagnosis for gout.

From Schumacher HR Jr (ed): *Primer on rheumatic diseases,* ed 9, Atlanta, 1988, Arthritis Foundation, p. 320.

VIII-12   CRITERIA FOR DIAGNOSIS OF PSORIATIC ARTHRITIS*

I. Mandatory
   A. Clinically apparent psoriasis (skin or nails) in association with pain and soft tissue swelling and/or limitation of motion in at least one joint, observed by a physician for 6 weeks or longer

II. Supportive
   A. Pain and soft tissue swelling and/or limitation of motion in one or more other joints, observed by a physician.
   B. Presence of an inflammatory arthritis in distal interphalangeal joint
   C. Specific exclusions—Heberden's or Bouchard's nodes
   D. Presence of "sausage" fingers or toes
   E. An asymmetric distribution of the arthritis in the hands and feet
   F. Absence of subcutaneous nodules
   G. A negative test for rheumatoid factor in the serum
   H. An inflammatory synovial fluid with a normal or increased C3 or C4 level, and an absence of (a) infection, including AFB, or (b) crystals of monosodium urate or calcium pyrophosphate
   I. A synovial biopsy showing synovial lining hypertrophy with a predominantly mononuclear cell infiltration and an absence of (a) granuloma formation or (b) tumor
   J. Peripheral radiographs showing an erosive arthritis of small joints with a relative lack of osteoporosis. Specific exclusion—erosive osteoarthritis

*Definite psoriatic arthritis—mandatory plus six supportive criteria. Probable psoriatic arthritis—mandatory plus four supportive criteria. Possible psoriatic arthritis—mandatory plus two supportive criteria.

From Bennett R. In McCarty DJ (ed): *Arthritis and allied conditions,* ed 11, Philadelphia, 1989, Lea & Febiger, p. 956.

VIII-13 DIFFERENTIAL DIAGNOSIS OF INFLAMMATORY MONOARTHRITIS

I. Crystal induced
   A. Gout
   B. Pseudogout
   C. Calcific tendinitis
II. Palindromic rheumatism
III. Infectious arthritis
   A. Septic
   B. Tubercular
   C. Fungal
   D. Viral
IV. Other
   A. Tendinitis
   B. Bursitis
   C. Juvenile rheumatoid arthritis

From McCarty D. In McCarty DJ (ed): *Arthritis and allied conditions*, ed 12, Philadelphia, 1993, Lea & Febiger, p.51.

VIII-14 DIAGNOSTIC FEATURES OF SARCOIDOSIS

I. Sarcoidosis
   A. Noncaseating granulomas on biopsy; must exclude other causes of granulomas
   B. Hilar and right paratracheal adenopathy in 90%
   C. Skin lesions, uveitis, or involvement of almost any tissue
   D. Onset most often in third and fourth decades, but cases reported at all ages.
   E. Impaired delayed hypersensitivity in 85%
   F. Frequent hyperglobulinemia
   G. Increased angiotensin-converting enzyme levels in about 80%.
   H. Hypercalciuria in most; hypercalcemia in some
II. Sarcoid arthropathy–acute sarcoidosis (Lofgren's syndrome, hilar adenopathy, fever, erythema nodosum)
   A. Often periarticular and very tender, warm swelling.
   B. Ankles and knees almost invariably involved.
   C. May be initial manifestation
   D. Joint motion may be normal
   E. Synovial effusions infrequent and usually mildly inflammatory when present
   F. Usually nonspecific mild synovitis on synovial biopsy
   G. Self-limited in weeks to 4 months
III. Chronic sarcoidosis
   A. May be acute and evanescent, recurrent, or chronic
   B. Noncaseating granulomas more commonly demonstrable in synovium
   C. Usually nondestructive despite chronic or recurrent disease

From Schumacher H. In McCarty DJ (ed): *Arthritis and allied conditions*, ed 12, Philadelphia, 1993, Lea & Febiger, pp. 1450-1452.

VIII-15   DIFFERENTIAL DIAGNOSIS OF POSITIVE BLOOD TEST FOR RHEUMATOID FACTOR

I. Rheumatologic disease
   A. Rheumatoid arthritis
   B. Juvenile rheumatoid arthritis
   C. Systemic lupus erythematosus
   D. Mixed connective tissue disease
   E. Behçet's syndrome
   F. Sjögren's syndrome
II. Infectious disease
   A. Bacterial (especially endocarditis)
   B. Syphilis
   C. Viral hepatitis
   D. Parasitic infections
   E. Granulomatous disease
   F. Mononucleosis
   G. AIDS
III. Pulmonary disease
   A. Bronchitis or asthma
   B. Coal miner's disease
   C. Asbestosis
   D. Idiopathic pulmonary fibrosis
   E. Sarcoidosis
IV. Other diseases
   A. Cirrhosis
   B. Myocardial infarction
   C. Neoplasms
   D. Essential mixed cryoglobulinemia
V. Healthy persons—increases with age

From Coffey R et al: *Postgraduate Medicine* 70:164, 1981.

VIII-16 CRYOGLOBULINEMIA

I. Essential or idiopathic
II. Secondary to or associated with
   A. Hemopoietic disorders
      1. Multiple myeloma
      2. Waldenström's macroglobulinemia
      3. Lymphatic leukemia, lymphosarcoma
      4. Polycythemia vera
      5. Sickle cell anemia
   B. Connective tissue disorders
      1. Systemic lupus erythematosus
      2. Syndrome of arthralgia, purpura, nephritis, and weakness
      3. Rheumatoid arthritis
      4. Ankylosing spondylitis
      5. Polyarteritis nodosa
      6. Sjögren's syndrome
      7. Thyroiditis
      8. Lymphoepithelial tumors of parotid gland
      9. Acute poststreptococcal glomerulonephritis
   C. Chronic infections
      1. Subacute bacterial endocarditis
      2. Visceral leishmaniasis (kala-azar)
      3. Syphilis
      4. Toxoplasmosis
      5. Leprosy
      6. Malaria
      7. Schistosomiasis
      8. Lyme disease
      9. HIV
   D. Others
      1. Chronic liver disease (cirrhosis, cholecystitis, chronic hepatitis (especially hepatitis C), gallbladder neoplasm)
      2. Skin disorders (porphyria cutanea tarda, pemphigus, erythrodermia)
      3. Acute myocardial infarction
      4. Infectious mononucleosis
      5. Ulcerative colitis
      6. Sarcoidosis
      7. Cytomegalovirus infection

From Hunder GG. In Schumacher HR (ed): *Primer on rheumatic diseases,* ed 10, Atlanta, 1993, Arthritis Foundation, p. 145.

VIII-17 CLASSIFICATION OF THE VASCULITIC SYNDROMES

I. Systemic necrotizing vasculitis
    A. Classic polyarteritis nodosa
    B. Allergic angiitis and granulomatosis of Churg-Strauss
    C. Polyangiitis overlap syndrome
II. Hypersensitivity vasculitis
    A. Exogenous stimuli proved or suspected
        1. Henoch-Schölein purpura
        2. Serum sickness and serum sickness-like reactions
        3. Other drug-induced vasculitides
        4. Vasculitis associated with infectious diseases
    B. Endogenous antigens likely involved
        1. Vasculitis associated with neoplasms
        2. Vasculitis associated with connective tissue diseases
        3. Vasculitis associated with other underlying diseases
        4. Vasculitis associated with congenital deficiencies of the complement system
III. Wegener's granulomatosis
IV. Giant cell arteritis
    A. Temporal arteritis
    B. Takayasu's arteritis
V. Other vasculitis syndromes
    A. Mucocutaneous lymph node syndrome (Kawasaki's disease)
    B. Isolated central nervous system vasculitis
    C. Thromboangiitis obliterans (Buerger's disease)
    D. Miscellaneous vasculitides

From Fauci AS. In Isselbacher KJ et al (eds): *Harrison's principles of internal medicine,* ed 13, New York, 1994, McGraw-Hill, p. 1671.

VIII-18 AUTOANTIBODIES IN RHEUMATIC DISEASES: DISEASE ASSOCIATIONS AND MOLECULAR IDENTIFICATION

Antibody to	Disease association (percent prevalence)
Native double-stranded DNA (dsDNA)	SLE (>50%)*
Histones	SLE (70%)
	Drug-induced SLE (>95%)
Sm (Smith)	SLE (30%)*
Nuclear RNP	SLE (30%)
Ro/SSA (ribonuclear protein)	Mixed connective tissue disease (>95%)
	SLE (35%)
	Sjögren's syndrome (60%)
	Complete congenital heart block (>85%)
	Subacute cutaneous LE (85%)
La/SSB	SLE (15%)
	Sjögren's syndrome (40%)
	Complete congenital heart block
Jo_1 (Histidyl-tRNA Synthetase)	Dermatomyositis/Polymyositis (25%)*
Scl_{70}	Scleroderma (20%)*
Centromere kinetochore	CREST (70% to 90%)
	Diffuse scleroderma (10% to 20%)
Antineutrophil cytoplasmic antibody (ANCA)	Wegener granulomatosis (>90%)
	Limited Wegener (60%)
	Other vasculitides (low)
Phospholipid (cardiolipid)	SLE (30% to 40%)
	Unexplained fetal death (10% to 15%), vascular occlusion

*Disease-specific.
From *Medical knowledge self-assessment program (IX),* Part B, Book 6, American College of Physicians, 1991, p. 571.

VIII-19   PUTATIVE ASSOCIATIONS OF CPPD CRYSTAL DEPOSITION (PSEUDOGOUT)

I. Group A (true association–high probability)
   A. Hyperparathyroidism
   B. Hemochromatosis
   C. Hemosiderosis
   D. Hypophosphatasia
   E. Hypomagnesemia
   F. Hypothyroidism
   G. Gout
   H. Neuropathic joints
   I. Aging
   J. Amyloidosis
   K. Trauma/surgery
   L. Familial hypocalciuric hypercalcemia

II. Group B (true association–modest probability)
   A. Hyperthyroidism
   B. Renal stone
   C. Ankylosing hyperostosis
   D. Ochronosis
   E. Wilson's disease
   F. Hemophilia arthritis

III. Group C (true association–unlikely)
   A. Diabetes mellitus
   B. Hypertension
   C. Mild azotemia
   D. Hyperuricemia
   E. Gynecomastia
   F. Inflammatory bowel disease
   G. Rheumatoid arthritis
   H. Paget's disease of bone
   I. Acromegaly

CPPD, Calcium pyrophosphate dihydrate.

From Ryan LM, McCarty DJ. In McCarty DJ (ed): *Arthritis and allied conditions,* ed 11, Philadelphia, 1989, Lea & Febiger, p. 1730.

VIII-20   SYNOVIAL FLUID CHARACTERISTICS

	Normal	Group I noninflammatory	Group II inflammatory	Group III septic
Gross appearance	Transparent, clear	Transparent, yellow	Opaque or translucent, yellow	Opaque, yellow to green
Viscosity	High	High	Low	Variable
White cells/mm$_3$	<200	<200	5,000 - 75,000	>50,000, often >100,000
Polymorphonuclear leukocytes	<25%	<25%	>50%	>75%
Culture	Negative	Negative	Negative	Often positive
Glucose (mg/dl)	Nearly equal to blood	Nearly equal to blood	>25, lower than blood	>50, lower than blood
Associated conditions		Degenerative joint disease	Rheumatoid arthritis	Bacterial infections
		Trauma	Connective tissue diseases (SLE, PSS, DM/PM)	Compromised immunity (disease or medication related)
		Neuropathic arthropathy	Ankylosing spondylitis	Other joint disease
		Hypertrophic osteoarthroplasty	Other seronegative spondyloarthropathies (psoriatic - arthritis, Reiter's syndrome, arthritis of chronic inflammatory bowel disease)	
		Pigmented villonodular synovitis	Crystal-induced synovitis (gout or pseudogout)	
		SLE	Acute rheumatic fever	
		Acute rheumatic fever		
		Erythema nodosum		

From McCarty DJ. In McCarty DJ (ed): *Arthritis and allied conditions*, ed 12, Philadelphia, 1993, Lea & Febiger, pp. 65, 68.

VIII-21   THE AMERICAN COLLEGE OF RHEUMATOLOGY 1990 CRITERIA FOR THE CLASSIFICATION OF FIBROMYALGIA*

I. History of widespread pain

   A. *Definition*: Pain is considered widespread when all of the following are present:

      1. Pain in the left side of the body

      2. Pain in the right side of the body

      3. Pain above the waist

      4. Pain below the waist

   B. In addition, axial skeletal pain (cervical spine or anterior chest or thoracic spine or low back) must be present.

   C. In this definition, shoulder and buttock pain is considered as pain for each involved side.

   D. "Low back" pain is considered lower segment pain.

II. Pain in 11 of 18 tender point sites on digital palpation.†

   A. *Definition:* Pain,‡ on digital palpation, must be present in at least 11 of the following 18 tender point sites:

      1. *Occiput:* Bilateral, at the suboccipital muscle insertions.

      2. *Low cervical:* Bilateral, at the anterior aspects of the intertransverse spaces at C5-C7.

      3. *Trapezius:* Bilateral, at the midpoint of the upper border.

      4. *Supraspinatus:* Bilateral, at origins, above the scapula spine near the medial border.

      5. *Second rib:* Bilateral, at the second costochondral junctions, just lateral to the junctions on upper surfaces.

      6. *Lateral epicondyle:* Bilateral, 2 cm distal to the epicondyles.

      7. *Gluteal:* Bilateral, in upper outer quadrants of buttocks in anterior fold of muscle.

      8. *Greater trochanter:* Bilateral, posterior to the trochanteric prominence.

      9. *Knee:* Bilateral, at the medial fat pad proximal to the joint line.

*For classification purposes, patients will be said to have fibromyalgia if both criteria are satisfied. Widespread pain must have been present for at least 3 months. The presence of a second clinical disorder does not exclude the diagnosis of fibromyalgia.

†Digital palpation should be performed with an approximate force of 4 kg.

‡For a tender point to be considered "positive" the subject must state that the palpation was painful. "Tender" is not to be considered "painful."

From Wolfe F et al: *Arthritis Rheumatism* 33(2):171, 1990.

VIII-22 PAINFUL DISORDERS AND DIAGNOSTIC MANEUVERS IN THE CERVICAL SPINE REGION

I. Disorders
  A. Rheumatic disease
    1. Fibromyalgia*
    2. Polymyalgia rheumatica*
    3. Degenerative disc and joint disease*
    4. Ankylosing spondylitis
    5. Peripheral spondyloarthropathies
    6. Crytan deposition disease
    7. Rheumatoid arthritis
    8. Diffuse idiopathic skeletal hyperostosis
  B. Regional cervical diseases
    1. Myofascial pain
    2. Osteomyelitis, septic arthritis or discitis
    3. Cervical lymphadenitis
    4. Thyroiditis
  C. Miscellaneous
    1. Thyroiditis
    2. Trauma-fractures
    3. Thoracic outlet syndrome
    4. Meningitis
    5. Osteoporosis
    6. Metastatic tumor
II. Diagnosis
  A. History
    1. Duration
    2. Pain related to motion
    3. Neurologic symptoms (numbness, paresthesia, weakness)
  B. Physical examination
    1. Spine tenderness
    2. Neck compression test (pain with flexing and compressing head)
    3. Axial manual traction test (pain relief with traction of head)
    4. Trigger points
    5. Neurologic deficits–abnormal DTRs (bicep, tricep), localized weakness
  C. Laboratory
    1. Routine radiography
    2. Computed tomography
    3. Magnetic resonance imaging
    4. Electromyography

*Most common.

CHAPTER IX

Neurology

IX-1 CLASSIFICATION OF COMA AND DIFFERENTIAL DIAGNOSIS

I. Diseases that cause no focal or lateralizing neurologic signs or alteration of the cellular content of the CSF. Usually brainstem functions and CT are normal
   A. Intoxications: alcohol, barbiturates, opiates, etc
   B. Metabolic disturbances: anoxia, diabetic acidosis, uremia, hepatic coma, hypoglycemia, Addisonian crisis, profound nutritional deficiency
   C. Severe systemic infections: pneumonia, typhoid fever, malaria, septicemia, Waterhouse-Friderichsen syndrome
   D. Circulatory collapse from any cause, and cardiac decompensation in the aged
   E. Epilepsy: postictal states
   F. Hypertensive encephalopathy and eclampsia
   G. Hyperthermia or hypothermia
   H. Concussion

II. Diseases that cause meningeal irritation with blood or an excess of white cells in the CSF, usually without focal or lateralizing cerebral or brainstem signs; CT or MRI scan may be normal or abnormal
   A. Subarachnoid hemorrhage from ruptured aneurysm, AV malformation, occasionally trauma
   B. Acute bacterial meningitis
   C. Some forms of viral encephalitis

III. Diseases that cause focal brainstem or lateralizing cerebral signs, with or without changes in the CSF, CT scan is usually abnormal
   A. Brain hemorrhage
   B. Cerebral infarction due to thrombosis or embolism
   C. Brain abscess, subdural empyema
   D. Epidural and subdural hemorrhage and brain contusion
   E. Brain tumor
   F. Miscellaneous: e.g., cortical vein thrombosis, some forms of viral encephalitis, focal embolic encephalomalacia due to bacterial endocarditis, acute hemorrhagic leukoencephalitis, disseminated (postinfectious) encephalomyelitis

From Adams R, Victor M: *Principles of neurology,* ed 5, New York, 1993, McGraw-Hill, pp. 312-313.

IX-2   DIFFERENTIAL DIAGNOSIS OF MENINGITIS

I. Bacterial meningitis
- A. *Neisseria meningitidis*
- B. *Haemophilus influenzae*
- C. *Streptococcus pneumoniae*
- D. *Staphylococcus aureus* and *S. epidermidis*
- E. Gram negative
  1. *Escherichia coli*
  2. Klebsiella, Proteus, Pseudomonas
- F. Mycobacteria
- G. Leptospirosis
- H. Rare
  1. *Listeria monocytogenes*
  2. Mima-Herellea

II. Viral (aseptic) meningitis
- A. Enteroviruses
  1. Coxsackie viruses
  2. Echo viruses
- B. Herpes simplex
  1. Meningitis or meningoencephalitis
- C. Cytomegalovirus
- D. Epstein-Barr virus
- E. Measles
- F. Mumps
- G. Influenza
- H. Varicella zoster
- I. Rubella
- J. Adenovirus

III. Nonviral agents that may cause encephalitis-aseptic meningitis syndromes
- A. Rickettsial
  1. Rocky Mountain spotted fever
  2. Q fever
- B. Chlamydia and mycoplasma
  1. Mycoplasma pneumoniae
  2. Psittacosis
- C. Mollaret recurrent meningitis
- D. Vogt-Koyanagi Harada syndrome
- E. NSAIDs

IX-3   DIFFERENTIAL DIAGNOSIS OF PERIPHERAL NEUROPATHIES*

I. *D*rugs (nitrofurantoin, INH, pyridoxine in excess, vincristine, etc)
II. *A*lcohol
III. *N*utritional (pernicious anemia, thiamine, B_6)
IV. *G*uillain-Barré syndrome
V. *T*oxins (heavy metals—arsenic, lead, etc.)
VI. *H*ereditary
VII. *E*ndocrine (diabetes mellitus, hypothyroidism)
VIII. *R*enal failure
IX. *A*myloidosis
X. *P*orphyria
XI. *I*nfections (syphilis, mononucleosis, diphtheria, leprosy)
XII. *S*ystemic disorders (rheumatoid arthritis, SLE, vasculitis, sarcoidosis)
XII. *T*umors

*Mnemonic to remember the classification: DANG THERAPIST.

From Griffin JW, Cornblath DR. In Harvey AM et al (eds): *The principles and practice of medicine*, ed 22, Norwalk, Conn, 1988, Appleton-Century-Crofts, p. 1093.

IX-4 CLASSIFICATION OF DEMENTIA

I. Diseases in which dementia is associated with clinical and laboratory signs of other medical disease.
   A. Hypothyroidism
   B. Cushing syndrome
   C. Nutritional deficiency states such as pellagra, the Wernicke-Korsakoff syndrome, and subacute combined degeneration of spinal cord and brain (vitamin B_{12} deficiency)
   D. Chronic meningoencephalitis: general paresis, meningovascular syphilis, cryptococcosis
   E. Hepatolenticular degeneration, familial and acquired
   F. Chronic drug intoxication
   G. AIDS

II. Diseases in which dementia is associated with other neurologic signs but not with other obvious medical disease
   A. Invariably associated with other neurologic signs
      1. Huntington chorea (choreoathetosis)
      2. Schilder disease and related demyelinative diseases (spastic weakness, pseudobulbar palsy, blindness)
      3. Amaurotic familial idiocy and other lipid-storage diseases (myoclonic seizures, blindness, spasticity, cerebellar ataxia)
      4. Myoclonic epilepsy (diffuse myoclonus, generalized seizures, cerebellar ataxia)
      5. Subacute spongiform encephalopathy or one type of Creutzfeldt-Jakob disease (myoclonic dementia)
      6. Cerebrocerebellar degeneration (cerebellar ataxia)
      7. Cerebral-basal ganglionic degenerations (apraxia-rigidity)
      8. Dementia with spastic paraplegia (spastic legs)
      9. Progressive supranuclear palsy
      10. Certain hereditary metabolic diseases
   B. Often associated with other neurologic signs
      1. Thrombotic or embolic cerebral infarction
      2. Brain tumor (primary or metastatic) or abscess
      3. Brain trauma, such as cerebral contusion, midbrain hemorrhage, chronic subdural hematoma
      4. Marchiafava-Bignami disease (often with apraxia and other frontal lobe signs)
      5. Communicating (normal-pressure) or obstructive hydrocephalus (usually with ataxia of gait)
      6. Progressive multifocal leukoencephalopathy

III. Diseases in which dementia is usually the only evidence of neurologic or medical disease
   A. Alzheimer disease
   B. Pick disease
   C. AIDS dementia
   D. Alcoholic dementia

From Adams R, Victor M: *Principles of neurology,* ed 5, New York, 1993, McGraw-Hill, p. 370.

IX-5   CLASSIFICATION OF DELIRIUM AND ACUTE CONFUSIONAL STATES

I. Delirium

    A. In a medical or surgical illness (no focal or lateralizing neurologic sign; CSF usually clear)

        1. Typhoid fever

        2. Pneumonia

        3. Septicemia, particularly erysipelas and other streptococcal infections

        4. Rheumatic fever

        5. Thyrotoxicosis and ACTH intoxication (rare)

        6. Postoperative and postconcussive states

    B. In neurologic disease that causes focal or lateralizing signs or changes in the CSF

        1. Vascular, neoplastic, or other diseases, particularly those involving the temporal and parietal lobes and upper part of the brainstem

        2. Cerebral contusion and laceration (traumatic delirium)

        3. Acute purulent and tuberculous meningitis

        4. Subarachnoid hemorrhage

        5. Encephalitis due to viral causes (e.g., herpes simplex, infectious mononucleosis) and to unknown causes

    C. The abstinence states, exogenous intoxications, and postconvulsive states; signs of other medical, surgical and neurologic illnesses absent or coincidental

        1. Withdrawal of alcohol (delirium tremens), barbiturates, and nonbarbiturate sedative drugs after chronic intoxication

        2. Drug intoxications: scopolamine, atropine, amphetamine, etc

        3. Postconvulsive delirium

Continued

IX-5 CLASSIFICATION OF DELIRIUM AND ACUTE CONFUSIONAL STATES—*cont'd*

II. Acute confusional states associated with psychomotor underactivity
  A. Associated with a medical or surgical disease (no focal or lateralizing neurologic signs; CSF clear)
    1. Metabolic disorders; hepatic stupor, uremia, hypoxia, hypercapnia, hypoglycemia, porphyria
    2. Infective fevers, especially typhoid
    3. Congestive heart failure
    4. Postoperative and posttraumatic psychoses
  B. Associated with drug intoxication (no focal or lateralizing signs; CSF clear): opiates, barbiturates and other sedatives, Artane, etc.
  C. Associated with diseases of the nervous system (with focal or lateralizing neurologic signs and/or CSF changes)
    1. Cerebral vascular disease, tumor, abscess
    2. Subdural hematoma
    3. Meningitis
    4. Encephalitis
III. Beclouded dementia, i.e., senile or other brain disease in combination with infective fevers, drug reactions, heart failure, or other medical or surgical diseases

From Adams R, Victor M: *Principles of neurology,* ed 5, New York, 1993, McGraw-Hill, p. 359.

IX-6   SECONDARY CAUSES OF DEPRESSION

I. Neurologic diseases
   A. Neuronal degenerations–Alzheimer's, Huntington's, and Parkinson's disease
   B. Focal CNS disease–strokes, brain tumors and trauma, and multiple sclerosis

II. Metabolic and endocrine diseases
   A. Corticosteroids, excess or deficiency
   B. Hypothyroidism, rarely thyrotoxicosis
   C. Cushing syndrome
   D. Addison's disease
   E. Hyperparathyroidism
   F. Pernicious anemia
   G. Chronic renal failure/dialysis
   H. B-vitamin deficiencies

III. Myocardial infarction, open heart surgery, and other operations

IV. Infectious diseases
   A. Brucellosis
   B. Viral hepatitis, influenza, pneumonia
   C. Infectious mononucleosis

V. Cancer, particularly pancreatic

VI. Parturition

VII. Medications
   A. Analgesics and antiinflammatory agents (other than steroids)–indomethacin, phenacetin, and phenylbutazone
   B. Amphetamines (when withdrawn)
   C. Antibiotics, particularly cycloserine, ethionamide, griseofulvin, isoniazid, nalidixic acid, and sulfonamides
   D. Antihypertensive drugs–clonidine, methyldopa, propranolol, reserpine
   E. Cardiac drugs–digitalis, procainamide
   F. Corticosteroids and ACTH
   G. Disulfiram
   H. L-Dopa
   I. Methysergide
   J. Oral contraceptives

From Adams R, Victor M: *Principles of neurology,* ed 5, New York, 1993, McGraw-Hill, p. 1314.

IX-7 CAUSES OF HYPOGLYCORRHACHIA (DECREASED CSF GLUCOSE)

   I. Pyogenic meningitis
  II. Tubercular meningitis
 III. Fungal meningitis
 IV. Sarcoidosis
  V. Subarachnoid hemorrhage (recent)
 VI. Meningeal carcinomatosis
VII. Occasional causes
    A. Mumps meningoencephalitis
    B. Herpes encephalitis
    C. Zoster encephalitis

From Adams R, Victor M: *Principles of neurology*, ed 4, New York, 1989, McGraw-Hill, p. 14.

IX-8   CAUSES OF HEADACHE

I. Extracranial
- A. Muscle contraction
- B. Cervical arthritis
- C. Sinusitis
- D. Glaucoma
- E. Otitis media
- F. Dental abscess
- G. Nasopharyngeal carcinoma
- H. Cranial arteritis

II. Intracranial
- A. Vascular
  1. Migraine
  2. Cluster
  3. Hypertension
  4. Subarachnoid hemorrhage
- B. Infection
  1. Meningitis
  2. Encephalitis
  3. Brain abscess
  4. Systemic infection
- C. Mass lesion
  1. Brain tumor
  2. Brain abscess
- D. Trauma
  1. Subdural hematoma
  2. Posttraumatic syndrome
- E. Facial pain
  1. Trigeminal neuralgia
  2. Glossopharyngeal neuralgia
  3. Atypical facial pain
- F. Other
  1. Pseudotumor cerebri
  2. Postspinal

From Speed III WG, McArthur JC. In Harvey AM et al (eds): *The principles and practice of medicine,* ed 22, Norwalk, Conn, 1988, Appleton-Century-Crofts, p. 1093.

IX-9 CAUSES OF ISCHEMIC STROKE

I. Thrombosis
  A. Atherosclerosis
  B. Arteritis
    1. Temporal arteritis
    2. Granulomatous arteritis
    3. Polyarteritis
    4. Wegener's granulomatosis
    5. Granulomatous arteritis of the great vessels (Takayasu's arteritis, syphilis)
  C. Dissections
    1. Carotid
    2. Vertebral
    3. Intracranial arteries at the base of the brain (spontaneous or traumatic)
  D. Hematologic disorders (polycythemia, sickle cell disease, thrombotic thrombocytopenic purpura)
  E. Cerebral mass effect compressing intracranial arteries
  F. Miscellaneous (Moyamoya disease, fibromuscular dysplasia, Binswanger's disease)
II. Vasoconstriction
  A. Cerebral vasospasm following subarachnoid hemorrhage
  B. Reversible cerebral vasoconstriction: Etiology unknown, after migraine, trauma, and eclampsia of pregnancy
III. Embolism
  A. Atherothrombotic arterial source
    1. Bifurcation of common carotid artery
    2. Carotid siphon
    3. Distal vertebral artery
    4. Aortic arch
  B. Cardiac source
    1. Structural heart disease
      a. Congenital: mitral valve prolapse, patent foramen ovale, etc.
      b. Acquired: following myocardial infarction, marantic vegetation, etc.
    2. Dysrhythmia: atrial fibrillation, sick sinus syndrome, etc.
    3. Infection: acute bacterial endocarditis
  C. Unknown source
    1. Healthy child or adult
    2. Associations
      a. Hypercoagulable state secondary to systemic disease
      b. Carcinoma (especially pancreatic)
      c. Eclampsia of pregnancy
      d. Oral contraceptives
      e. Lupus
      f. Anticoagulants
      g. Factor C deficiency
      h. Factor S deficiency
      i. Factor V Leiden
      j. Phospholipid antibody syndrome

From Kistler JP, Ropper AH, Martin JB. In Isselbacher KJ et al (eds): *Harrison's principles of internal medicine*, ed 13, New York, 1994, McGraw-Hill, p. 2234.

CHAPTER X

Dermatology

X-1   CONDITIONS ASSOCIATED WITH ERYTHEMA NODOSUM

I. Drugs
   A. Estrogens
   B. Oral contraceptives
   C. Sulfonamides
   D. Aminopyrine*
   E. Antimony compounds*
   F. Arsphenamine*
   G. Bromides*
   H. Immunizations*
   I. Iodides*
   J. Phenacetin*
   K. Salicylates*
   L. Vaccines*
   M. Nitrofurantoin
   N. Trimethoprim

II. Infections
   A. Bacterial
      1. Streptococcal infection
      2. Tuberculosis
      3. Yersinia (Pasteurella) infection (especially Scandinavia), *Y. enterocolitica* and *Y. pseudotuberculosis*
      4. Brucellosis*
      5. Leptospirosis*
      6. Tularemia*
      7. Salmonellosis
      8. Campylobacter infection
      9. *Corynebacterium diphtheriae*
      10. Chancroid
      11. Meningococcal
      12. Atypical mycobacterial
   B. Chlamydial
   C. Fungal
      1. Coccidioidomycosis
      2. Histoplasmosis
      3. Dermatophytosis*
      4. North American blastomycosis*
      5. Sporotrichosis
   D. Protozoan:
      1. Toxoplasmosis
      2. Hookworm infection
   E. Viral
      1. Herpes simplex
      2. Infectious mononucleosis
      3. Milker's nodule
      4. Hepatitis

Continued

X-1   CONDITIONS ASSOCIATED WITH ERYTHEMA NODOSUM—*cont'd*

III. Malignancy*:
  A. Hodgkin's disease
  B. Leukemia
  C. Postradiated pelvic cancer
IV. Miscellaneous:
  A. Behçet's disease
  B. Inflammatory bowel disease (Crohn's disease, ulcerative colitis)
  C. Pregnancy*
  D. Sarcoidosis
  E. Reiter's disease

*Rare.

From White JW Jr, Hurley H. In Moschella S, Hurley H (eds): *Dermatology*, ed 3, Philadelphia, 1992, WB Saunders, p. 585.

X-2   CAUSES OF ANHIDROSIS

I. Neuropathic
  A. Hysteria
  B. Diseases or tumors of:
    1. Hypothalamus
    2. Pons
    3. Medulla
    4. Spinal cord
    5. Sympathetic nerves
II. Sweat gland disturbances
  A. Congenital defects
    1. Generalized
    2. Localized
  B. Acquired defects
    1. Dermal diseases
    2. Drugs—anticholinergics
    3. Toxic chemicals
  C. Obstruction of sweat ducts
    1. Inflammatory or keratotic dermatoses
    2. Miliaria
III. Idiopathic or indeterminate
  A. Newborn
  B. Local radiant heat or pressure
  C. Toxic
  D. Dehydration
  E. Systemic disease
  F. Franceschetti-Jadassohn syndrome
  G. Helweg-Larssen syndrome
  H. Fabry's disease

From Hurley H. In Moschella S, Hurley H (eds): *Dermatology*, ed 3, Philadelphia, 1992, WB Saunders, p. 1524

X-3   SUSPECTED ETIOLOGIC FACTORS IN ERYTHEMA MULTIFORME

I. Infections
   A. Viral
      1. Herpes simplex
      2. Infectious mononucleosis
      3. Vaccinia
   B. Bacterial
      1. Hemolytic streptococci
      2. Proteus
      3. Salmonella
      4. Staphylococcus
      5. Tuberculosis
      6. Tularemia
      7. *Vibrio parahaemolyticus*
      8. Yersinia
      9. *Mycoplasma pneumoniae*
   C. Fungal infections (histoplasmosis)
II. Drugs
   A. Allopurinol
   B. Antituberculous drugs (rifampin, isoniazid, thiacetazone).
   C. Barbiturates
   D. Carbamazepine
   E. Hydantoins
   F. NSAIDs (benoxaprofen, ibuprofen, fenoprofen, phenylbutazone)
   G. Sulfonamides (including hypoglycemics)
III. Neoplasia
IV. Physical factors
   A. Sunlight
   B. X-ray therapy
V. Endocrine factors (pregnancy)
VI. Collagen diseases and vasculitides
VII. Contact reactions (fire sponge [*Tedania ignis*])

From Elias P, Fritsch P. In Fitzpatrick TB et al (eds): *Dermatology in general medicine,* ed 4, New York, 1993 McGraw-Hill, p. 587.

X-4 CLINICAL MANIFESTATIONS OF MASTOCYTOSIS

I. Cutaneous
   A. Reddish-brown papules
   B. Flush
II. Cardiovascular
   A. Tachycardia, hypotension, and syncope (rarely fatal)
III. Gastrointestinal
   A. Nausea, vomiting, diarrhea (exacerbated by alcohol)
   B. Malabsorption (rare)
   C. Portal hypertension (rare)
IV. Bone
   A. Pain
V. Neurologic
   A. Neuropsychiatric symptoms (malaise, irritability)
VI. Respiratory
   A. Rhinorrhea, wheezing (rare)
VII. Hematologic
   A. Anemia, leukopenia, thrombocytopenia (rare)
   B. Eosinophilia
   C. Coagulopathies
   D. Leukemia (rare)

From Lewis R, Austen K. In Fitzpatrick TB et al (eds): *Dermatology in general medicine,* ed 3, New York, 1987, McGraw-Hill, p. 1900.

X-5   CLASSIFICATION OF CUTANEOUS SIGNS OF INTERNAL MALIGNANCY

I. Lesions secondary to the deposition of substances in the skin
   A. Icterus
   B. Melanosis
   C. Hemochromatosis
   D. Xanthomas
   E. Systemic amyloidosis
II. Vascular and blood abnormalities
   A. Flushing
   B. Palmar erythema
   C. Telangiectasia
   D. Purpura
   E. Vasculitis
   F. Cutaneous ischemia
   G. Thrombophlebitis
III. Bullous disorders
   A. Bullous pemphigoid
   B. Pemphigus vulgaris
   C. Dermatitis herpetiformis
   D. Herpes gestationis
   E. Erythema multiforme
   F. Epidermolysis bullosa acquisita
   G. Linear IgA dermatosis
IV. Infections and manifestations
   A. Herpes zoster
   B. Herpes simplex
   C. Bacterial infections
   D. Fungi and yeast infections
   E. Scabies
V. Disorders of keratinization
   *A. Acanthosis nigricans
   B. Acquired ichthyosis
   C. Palmar hyperkeratosis
   D. Erythroderma
   *E. Paraneoplastic acrokeratosis of Bazex
VI. Collagen-vascular disease
   A. Dermatomyositis
   B. Lupus erythematosus
   C. Progressive systemic sclerosis
VII. Skin tumors and internal malignant disease
   A. Muir-Torre syndrome
   B. Gardner's syndrome
   C. Cowden's disease
   D. Mucosal neuroma syndrome
   E. Neurofibromatosis

Continued

X-5 CLASSIFICATION OF CUTANEOUS SIGNS OF INTERNAL MALIGNANCY—*cont'd*

VIII. Hormone-related conditions

IX. Disorders associated with primary skin cancer
  A. Nevoid basal cell carcinoma syndrome
  B. Arsenical manifestations

X. Various disorders associated with internal malignant disease
  A. Pruritus
  *B. Erythema gyratum repens
  C. Subcutaneous fat necrosis
  *D. Sweet's syndrome
  *E. Hypertrichosis lanuginosa acquisita
  *F. Necrolytic migratory erythema
  G. Clubbing
  H. Leukoderma
  I. Peutz-Jeghers syndrome
  J. Tuberous sclerosis
  K. Wiskott-Aldrich syndrome
  L. Multiple eruptive seborrheic keratoses
  M. Porphyria cutanea tarda
  *N. Paget's disease

XI. Direct tumor involvement in the skin

*Definite associations.

From Mclean DI, Haynes HA. In *Dermatology in general medicine,* Fitzpatrick TB et al (eds): ed 4, New York, 1993, McGraw-Hill, p. 2229.

X-6 DRUGS THAT CAUSE PRURITUS

I. Opiates and derivatives
  A. Cocaine
  B. Morphine
  C. Butorphanol

II. Via cholestasis
  A. Phenothiazines
  B. Tolbutamide
  C. Erythromycin estolate
  D. Anabolic hormones
  E. Estrogens
  F. Progestins
  G. Testosterone

III. Aspirin

IV. Quinidine

V. Vitamin B complex

VI. Psoralen + UVA radiation (PUVA)

VII. Subclinical sensitivity to any drug

From Bernard J. In Fitzpatrick TB et al (eds): *Dermatology in general medicine,* ed 3, New York, 1987, McGraw-Hill, p. 81.

X-7 COMMON SKIN DISORDERS IN THE ELDERLY

I. Dermatoses
  A. Dermatoheliosis (photoaging)
  B. Pruritus
  C. Xerosis and eczema craquelé
  D. Neurodermatitis
  E: Statis dermatitis and ulceration
  F. Nummular dermatitis
  G. Persistent contact dermatitis
  H. Seborrheic dermatitis
  I. Granuloma fissuratum
  J. Angular cheilitis
  K. Chondrodermatitis nodular helicis
  L. Bullous pemphigoid
  M. Decubitus ulceration
  N. Calluses and corns
  O. Drug reactions
II. Infections and infestations
  A. Tinea pedis/tinea unguium
  B. Herpes zoster (shingles)
  C. Intertrigo
  D. Scabies
III. Neoplasms
  A. Acrochordons (skin tags)
  B. Seborrheic keratoses
  C. Cherry hemangiomas
  D. Sebaceous hyperplasia
  E. Actinic keratoses
  F. Basal cell carcinoma
  G. Squamous cell carcinoma
  H. Lentigo maligna
  I. Lentigo maligna melanoma
  J. Cutaneous T cell lymphoma (mycosis fungoides)

From Fenske NA, Lober CW. In Moschella S, Hurley H (eds): *Dermatology*, ed 3, Philadelphia, 1992, WB Saunders, p. 108.

CHAPTER XI

Acquired Immunodeficiency Syndrome (AIDS)

XI-1   CLASSIFICATION SYSTEM FOR HIV INFECTION

	Clinical categories		
CD4+ T-cell categories	(A)† Asymptomatic, acute HIV or PGL*	(B)† Symptomatic, not (A) or (C) conditions	(C)† AIDS-indicator conditions
(1) >/=500	A1	B1	C1
(2) 200-449	A2	B2	C2
(3) <200 Aids Indicator T-cell count	A3	B3	C3

*PGl, Persistent generalized lymphadenopathy.

†See following text for discussion:

Category B consists of symptomatic conditions in an HIV-infected individual that are not included among conditions listed in Category C and that meet at least one of the following criteris: a) the conditions are attributed to HIV infection or are indicative of a defect in cell-mediated immunity; or b) the conditions are considered by physicians to have a clinical course or to require management that is complicated by HIV infection. *Examples* include (but are not limited to) Bacillary angiomatosis; Oropharyngeal candidiasis; Oral hairy leukoplakia; Herpes zoster involving at least two distinct episodes or more than one dermatome; Listeriosis; Peripheral neuropathy; Candidiasis, vulvogaginal: persistent, frequent, or poorly responsive to therapy; Cervical dysplasia (moderate or severe)/cervical carcinoma in situ; Idiopathic thrombocytopenic purpura; Pelvic inflammatory disease. *Category C* includes Candidiasis of bronchi, trachea, or lungs; Esophageal candidiasis; Cervical cancer, invasive; Coccidiomycosis, extrapulmonary; Cryptosporidiosis, chronic intestinal; Cytomegalovirus disease (other than liver, spleen or nodes); Cytomegalovirus retinitis; Encephalopathy, HIV- related; Herpes simplex: chronic ulcer (>1 month duration); or bronchitis, pneumonitis, or esophagitis; Histoplasmosis, extrapulmonary; Isosporiasis, chronic intestinal; Kaposi's sarcoma; Lymphoma, Burkitt's; Lymphoma, immunoblastic; Lymphoma, brain primary; *M. avium* complex or *M. kansasii,* extrapulmonary; *M. tuberculosis,* any site (pulmonary or extrapulmonary); *Mycobacterium,* other species, extrapulmonary; *Pneumocystis carinii* pneumonia; Pneumonia, recurrent; Progressive multifocal leukoencephalopathy; *Salmonella* septicemia, recurrent; Toxoplasmosis of the brain; Wasting syndrome due to HIV.

From CDC: *MMWR* 41 (No. RR-17):2-4, 1992.

XI-2   RELATION OF CLINICAL MANIFESTATIONS TO CD4 COUNT IN HIV-INFECTED PATIENTS

	Circulating CD4 count at time of initial susceptibility			
	>500	500-200	<200	<50
Asymptomatic	•			
Kaposi's sarcoma	•			
Fever, sweats, weight loss		•		
Hairy leukoplakia		•		
Oral, esophageal candida		•		
Tuberculosis		•		
Pneumocystosis			•	
Cryptococcosis			•	
Dementia			•	
Toxoplasmosis				•
Mycobacterium A/I				•
CMV				•
Death				•

From Shelhamer JH et al: *Ann Intern Med* 117(5):419, 1992.

XI-3   RENAL SYNDROMES IN PATIENTS WITH HIV INFECTION

I. Coincidental renal syndromes and HIV
   A. Acute renal failure (ARF)
      1. Acute tubular necrosis from hypovolemic, anoxic, and toxic injuries
      2. Allergic interstitial nephritis from drugs
      3. Azotemia from nonsteroidal antiinflammatory drugs
      4. Renal failure from massive proteinuria and severe hypoalbuminemia (intrarenal edema)
      5. Postinfectious immune complex glomerulonephritis
      6. Sulfadiazine and acyclovir crystal induced renal failure
      7. Plasmacytic interstitial nephritis
      8. Hemolytic uremic syndrome
   B. Acid-base and fluid-electrolyte derangements
      1. Hyponatremia and hypernatremia
      2. Inappropriate secretion of antidiuretic hormone (ADH)
      3. Hypokalemia and hyperkalemia
      4. Type IV renal tubular acidosis (hyporeninemic hypoaldosteronism)
      5. Metabolic alkalosis
      6. Hypomagnesemia
      7. Hypouricemia
   C. Infections in the kidney
      1. Microabscesses from bacterial infections *(Staphylococcus aureus)*
      2. Tuberculosis of the kidney (both typical and atypical mycobacterium)
      3. Cytomegalovirus infection
      4. Candida, cryptococcal, aspergillus, and other fungal infections
   D. Infiltrations in the kidney
      1. Lymphoma of the kidney
      2. Kaposi's sarcoma
      3. Amyloidosis of the kidney
      4. Calcifications of the kidney

II. Specific (?) renal disorder; HIV-associated nephropathy
   A. Focal and segmental glomerulosclerosis
   B. Other forms of glomerulonephritis

III. Renal disease occurring in HIV seropositive patients
   A. Heroin-associated nephropathy
   B. Diabetic glomerulosclerosis, polycystic kidney disease, etc.
   C. Obstructive uropathy

IV. Superimposed HIV infection in those with renal replacement therapy
   A. Maintenance dialysis patients acquiring HIV from blood transfusions, intravenous drug abuse, and sexual contacts
   B. Renal transplant recipients developing HIV infection through renal allograft, blood transfusions, intravenous drug abuse, and sexual contacts

From Rao TK: *Ann Rev Med* 42:391-401, 1991

XI-4 MAJOR ENDOCRINE COMPLICATIONS IN ACQUIRED IMMUNODEFICIENCY SYNDROME

Gland	Complication	Most likely causes
Adrenal	Cortisol and aldosterone deficiency	Opportunistic infection or ketoconazole
Pituitary	Syndrome of inappropriate anti-diuretic hormone (SIADH)	Pulmonary or central nervous system infection or drugs
Thyroid	Euthyroid sick	Systemic illness
Pancreatic islets	Hypoglycemia	Pentamidine, inanition, or sepsis
Testis	Hypogonadism	Hypothalamic deficiency secondary to systemic illness or ketoconazole
	Gynecomastia	Ketoconazole
Parathyroid	Hypocalcemia	Systemic illness or hypomagnesemia

From Aron DC: *Arch Intern Med* 149:330, 1989.

XI-5   GASTROINTESTINAL MANIFESTATIONS OF AIDS

I. Mouth
   A. Candidiasis
   B. Aphthous ulcers
   C. Hairy leukoplakia
   D. Acute necrotizing ulcerative gingivitis

II. Esophagus
   A. Candidiasis
   B. CMV infection
   C. Herpes simplex
   D. Mycobacterial infection
   E. Fungal infection (histoplasmosis, coccidiomycosis)

III. Liver and biliary tree
   A. Viral hepatitis (types A, B, and C)
   B. Chronic active hepatitis
   C. CMV hepatitis
   D. Hepatic granulomas (e.g., fungal, drug-induced)
   E. Alcoholic hepatitis
   F. Steatosis
   G. Sclerosing cholangitis (CMV, cryptosporidiosis)
   H. Ampullary stenosis

IV. Small bowel
   A. CMV infection
   B. Cryptosporidiosis
   C. Giardiasis
   D. *Isopora belli* infection
   E. Microsporidiosis
   F. MAI infection
   G. "AIDS enteropathy"
   H. Enteropathogenic bacterial infection
   I. Antibiotic-associated colitis
   J. Bacterial enteritides (Salmonella, Shigella)

V. Acute pancreatitis
   A. Medications (TMP/SMX, pentamidine, ddl)

VI. Neoplasms
   A. Kaposi's sarcoma
   B. Lymphoma

XI-6 GASTROINTESTINAL PATHOGENS IN HIV-INFECTED PATIENTS*

Organ	Pathogens
Esophagus	*Candida albicans;* herpes simplex virus; cytomegalovirus
Stomach	Cytomegalovirus; *Mycobacterium avium-intracellulare*
Small intestine	*Cryptosporidium; Microsporidium; Isospora belli; Mycobacterium avium-intracellulare; Salmonella* species; *Campylobacter jejuni*
Colon	Cytomegalovirus; *Chlamydia trachomatis; Cryptosporidium; Mycobacterium avium-intracellulare;* amebiasis; candidiasis; *Shigella flexneri; Clostridium difficile; Campylobacter jejuni; Histoplasma capsulatum;* adenovirus; herpes simplex virus (rectum); gonorrhea (proctitis); syphilis (proctitis)

*HIV, Human immunodeficiency virus.
From Smith PD et al: *Ann Intern Med* 116(1):64, 1992.

XI-7 RHEUMATOLOGIC MANIFESTATIONS OF INFECTION WITH HUMAN IMMUNODEFICIENCY VIRUS (HIV)

I. Arthritis
   A. Reiter syndrome and other reactive arthritides
   B. Psoriatic arthritis
   C. Septic arthritis caused by opportunistic organisms
   D. HIV-associated arthritis
II. Arthralgia
III. Myopathies
   A. Polymyositis
   B. Zidovudine-induced myositis
   C. Necrotizing, noninflammatory myopathy
   D. Pyomyositis
   E. Infectious myositis with opportunistic organisms
   F. Nemaline (rod) myopathy
   G. Myositis ossificans
   H. Subclinical myopathy
IV. Vasculitis
   A. Necrotizing vasculitis
   B. Eosinophilic vasculitis
   C. Isolated granulomatous angiitis of the central nervous system
   D. Leukocytoclastic vasculitis
   E. Lymphomatoid granulomatosis
   F. The sicca syndrome

From Kaye BR: *Ann Intern Med* 111(2):159, 1989.

XI-8 AIDS-ASSOCIATED HEMATOLOGIC DISORDERS

I. Anemia (70%)
   A. Marrow infiltration
      1. Infection: MAI, CMV, cryptococcus, histoplasmosis
      2. Lymphoma
   B. GI blood loss (Kaposi's sarcoma)
   C. Antierythrocyte antibodies (especially anti-i)
   D. Myelosuppression due to drugs: AZT, gancyclovir, pentamidine, Bactrim, acyclovir

II. Thrombocytopenia (40%)
   A. Immune-mediated destruction (ITP)
   B. Impaired synthesis—marrow infiltration
   C. HUS/TTP-like syndromes
   D. Drugs: e.g., AZT

III. Granulocytopenia (50%)

IV. Lymphopenic (70%)

V. Coagulation abnormalities
   A. Antiphospholipid antibody with elevated PTT

From Scadden D, Zon L, Groopman J: *Blood* 74(5):1455-1461, October 1989.

XI-9 MUCOCUTANEOUS MANIFESTATIONS IN AIDS

I. Skin
   A. Infections
      1. Exaggerated scabies
      2. Herpes zoster (dermatomal or disseminated)
      3. Molluscum contagiosum
      4. Herpes simplex
      5. Dermatophytosis
      6. Cat-scratch disease
      7. Cutaneous cryptococcosis
   B. Granuloma annulare
   C. Kaposi's sarcoma
   D. Psoriatic exacerbation
   E. Inflammatory seborrheic dermatitis
   F. Ichthyosis
   G. Xerosis
   H. Papulonodular demodicidosis
   I. Bacillary epithelial angiomatosis
II. Hair
   A. Alopecia areata
   B. AIDS trichopathy
III. Nails
   A. Yellow nail syndrome
   B. Purple nail bands due to AZT
IV. Mouth
   A. Thrush
   B. Kaposi's sarcoma
   C. Hairy leukoplakia

From Orkin M, Maibach HE, Dahl MV: *Dermatology*, Norwalk, Conn, 1991, Appleton & Lange, p.145.

XI-10 PULMONARY COMPLICATIONS OF HIV INFECTION

I. Infections
- A. Viruses
  1. Cytomegalovirus
  2. Herpes simplex virus
  3. Varicella-zoster virus
  4. Epstein-Barr virus?
  5. Human immunodeficiency virus?
- B. Bacteria
  1. Pyogenic organisms (especially *Streptococcus pneumoniae, Haemophilus influenzae*)
  2. *Mycobacterium tuberculosis*
  3. *Mycobacterium avium* complex
  4. Other nontuberculous mycobacteria
  5. *Rhodococcus equi*
- C. Fungi
  1. Histoplasma capsulatum
  2. Coccidioides immitis
  3. Cryptococcus neoformans
  4. *Candida* species
  5. *Aspergillus* species
- D. Parasites
  1. *Pneumocystis carinii*
  2. *Toxoplasma gondii*
  3. *Cryptosporidium* species
  4. *Strongyloides stercoralis*

V. Malignancies
- A. Kaposi's sarcoma
- B. Non-Hodgkin's lymphoma

VI. Interstitial pneumonias
- A. Lymphocytic interstitial pneumonitis
- B. Nonspecific interstitial pneumonitis
- C. Drug-induced reactions

VII. Other
- A. Adult respiratory distress syndrome
- B. Secondary alveolar proteinosis

From Murray J, Mills J: *Am Rev Respir Dis* 141:1357, 1990.

XI-11 NEUROLOGIC PROBLEMS IN AIDS PATIENTS

I. Infectious
  A. Central nervous system
    1. Toxoplasmosis*
    2. Cryptococcosis*
    3. Herpes simplex*
    4. Cytomegalovirus *
    5. Neurosyphilis
    6. Progressive multifocal leukoencephalopathy*
    7. Candidiasis*
    8. Tuberculosis*
    9. Mycobacterium avium-intracellulare
    10. Varicella-zoster encephalitis
    11. Narcardiosis*
    12. Coccidiomycosis
  B. Peripheral nervous system
    1. Herpes zoster
    2. Cytomegalovirus polyradiculopathy
    3. HIV polyneuritis
II. Noninfectious
  A. Central nervous system
    1. HIV dementia
    2. Vacuolar myelopathy
    3. Lymphoma*
    4. Kaposi's sarcoma*
    5. Nonspecific gliosis*
  B. Peripheral nervous system
    1. Sensory neuropathy
    2. Inflammatory demyelinating neuropathy
    3. Mononeuritis multiplex
    4. Polymyositis and other myopathies
III. Psychiatric
  A. Depression
  B. Anxiety-panic disorder
  C. Delirium
  D. Mania
  E. Psychosis

*May cause intracranial mass lesion.

XI-12   CANCERS IN THE HIV EPIDEMIC

I. Incidence increased:
   A. Kaposi's sarcoma
   B. CNS non-Hodgkin's lymphoma
   C. Peripheral non-Hodgkin's lymphoma
   D. Cervical carcinoma
II. Cases reported
   A. Hodgkin's lymphoma
   B. Squamous carcinoma
   C. Small cell carcinoma
   D. Testicular cancer
   E. Basal cell cancer
   F. Melanoma
III. Anticipated relationship:
   A. Hepatocellular carcinoma

From Chaisson R, Volberding P. Clinical manifestations of HIV infection. In Mandell GL et al (eds): *Principles and practice of infectious diseases,* ed 4, Churchill Livingstone, 1995, New York, p. 1245.

XI-13 CLINICAL MANIFESTATIONS OF PRIMARY HIV INFECTION

I. General
   A. Fever
   B. Pharyngitis
   C. Lymphadenopathy
   D. Arthralgia
   E. Myalgia
   F. Lethargy/malaise
   G. Anorexia/weight loss

II. Neuropathic
   A. Headache
   B. Meningoencephalitis
   C. Peripheral neuropathy
   D. Radiculopathy
   E. Brachial neuritis
   F. Guillain-Barré syndrome
   G. Cognitive/affective impairment

III. Dermatologic
   A. Erythematous maculopapular rash
   B. Roseola-like rash
   C. Diffuse urticaria
   D. Desquamation
   E. Alopecia
   F. Mucocutaneous ulceration

IV. Gastrointestinal
   A. Oropharyngeal candidiasis
   B. Nausea/vomiting
   C. Diarrhea

V. Respiratory
   A. Cough

From Tindall B, Carr A, Cooper DA. In Sande MA, Volberding PA (eds): *The medical management of AIDS,* ed 4, Philadelphia, 1995, WB Saunders, p. 107.

Index